The

Salicylate

Handbook

The Salicylate Handbook

Your guide to understanding
salicylate sensitivity

Sharla Race

The Salicylate Handbook:
Your guide to understanding salicylate sensitivity

The original Salicylate Handbook was published in 2002 as an eBook in PDF format. This new, revised, edition is available in various formats.

First paperback edition
Published 2012
ISBN: 978-1-907119-04-0

Publisher: Tigmor Books
www.tigmorbooks.co.uk

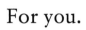

For you.

Contents

Welcome

My life before I knew I was salicylate sensitive was confusing, frustrating, and painful. Even as a child, I never seemed to be well and the doctors could rarely find anything wrong with me. Diagnoses changed over the years from growing pains, rheumatic fever, "just accident prone", to viral infection, post viral syndrome, stress, over work, over weight and so on. I am sure the underlying diagnosis was often "hypochondria" but nobody actually said that.

By the time, I was in my mid thirties I was a physical, mental and emotional wreck. Nothing I tried seemed to help. A healthy diet full of fruit and vegetables made me feel worse. Strict low calorie diets brought about some weight loss, usually not for long, but my other symptoms persisted. Counselling sorted out some of my inner confusion but changed nothing else. Homeopathy did help relieve some of my symptoms, especially the sinusitis, but the majority of the problems continued to recur.

My health deteriorated to such an extent that I was no longer able to go out to work. I had so little physical energy that even the simplest of tasks, such as feeding the cats, could reduce me to tears. My joints were stiff and inflexible making walking up stairs a nightmare. The additional muscle pain made lying down and sitting just as uncomfortable. I seemed to have a permanent headache, sometimes a migraine. My ears buzzed, my sinuses swam, my vision blurred, I put on weight and was bloated all the time.

Far worse than the physical symptoms was the loss of zest and interest in life. My memory was appalling and I felt confused, irritable and very scared. At first I had no energy to resist being so ill and did little else than sleep and watch television. This "inert" time was not wholly without some positives. The one thing I could do was think— yes, it was often muddled but I could still do it.

I had tried everything—the doctors said nothing was wrong, alternative therapies and miracle cure diets (and, believe me, I had tried them all) had not worked. Instinctively, I felt that there was nothing seriously wrong with me, that the answer to my problems did exist and that it was simple. I was missing something and I had to find out what it was. I was not going to spend the rest of my life in this state.

A short while before becoming very ill I had helped Alex, my husband, identify the cause of his migraines, high blood pressure and depression. As I watched him get thinner, healthier, and migraine and depression free, I started to muse on food intolerance. The links between food and migraines are well known, and accepted, which is why I had been insistent that he try various diets until we unravelled his problems—a tyramine sensitivity and yeast intolerance.

At the time, it never occurred to me that my own problems might also be related to food intolerance. In all honesty, my symptoms seemed so diverse that it just seemed a ridiculous idea. However, I had tried everything else. To say I was sceptical is a gross understatement of how I felt. I was simply going to try this avenue because I had reached a dead end down all the others.

It was not a straightforward process but I eventually discovered that all my problems were being caused by a sensitivity to salicylates. Finding the information I needed was exceedingly difficult as there is very little information readily available on salicylates, and a salicylate sensitivity, except in respect of aspirin, is not accepted by many doctors. I persevered and eventually was able to pull together enough information to begin my healing process.

I would be misleading you if I was to say everything changed overnight. Some things did. Suddenly I had more energy, my skin was clearer, my muscles and joints stopped hurting, I began to sleep better, felt calmer, stopped having mood swings, no longer experienced anxiety, lost weight, and so on. If only that could have been the end of the story but, sadly, it wasn't.

After a period of amazing good health, I began to experience the same problems when exposed to perfumes, air fresheners, detergents, scented candles, glues, paints and, so it seemed, virtually anything that had a smell and some things that didn't. I began to suspect that I had developed full-blown Multiple Chemical Sensitivity. Going anywhere outside of the house led to a reaction that left me ill for days. I seemed to get over one reaction and then another would arrive.

Bewildered, I delved back into more research and discovered that salicylate not only occurs naturally in food but also, in various other forms, is used in the manufacture of the products that we use every day in our homes, shops, and offices. I had already discovered that applying a product containing salicylate on my skin would lead to problems (chemical like burns on my face and scalp after using a highly coloured shampoo, a blotchy rash from a soap scented with oil of wintergreen and so on). Perhaps the same applied to inhaled salicylate. We cleared the house of as many scented products and chemicals as possible and tried to cut down on my exposure outside of the home. Almost imperceptibly, the changes began to take place. I began to have fewer reactions and the severity of the ones I had began to reduce.

I still experience reactions but, generally, only away from the home. My activities are restricted but less so than when I was ill—at least now I can walk pain free and think clearly! The freedom and relief that I now have from simply being able to understand what was causing my problems is immense and extremely liberating. I no longer have to waste time worrying about what is wrong with me—I know and as long as I control my diet and limit my inhaled exposures, I am healthy.

Convinced that I was far from unique, I wanted to share my experiences and the information I had acquired and so the *Food Can Make You Ill* (www.foodcanmakeyouill.co.uk) web site was born. That and the success of my first book, *Change Your Diet and Change Your Life*, further fuelled my drive to get information on food intolerance out to people. If my life could be so impaired so could that of others. If I could experience such dramatic changes, physically, mentally and emotionally, then so could others.

I have resisted writing *The Salicylate Handbook* for some time because I still feel as if I am learning but as the number of queries I receive on salicylate continuously increases I felt that the time was right to pull together the knowledge that I had acquired and to share it with others.

You should be aware that the role of salicylate in illness is a controversial one and is not accepted by many in the medical profession. I hope that in time this will change and the hidden suffering that many undergo will stop but until that time we have to do the best we can with the information we have available. This handbook is designed to be used as a resource you can dip into whenever you need to check on the different ways in which salicylate sensitivity can affect your health. Before using it in this way, I suggest you familiarise yourself with the whole book.

Wherever possible, I have included references so that you can follow up specific papers of interest. I have endeavoured to keep the amount of scientific jargon to a bare minimum and have only used studies that I have been able to "translate". My own experience is interwoven throughout and I make no apology for the speculation that also appears.

The above is the original 2002 introduction. So, has anything changed in the last ten years?

There have been some new studies on salicylate levels in food but they have been limited in scope and added very little to what we already know. I have however gone through these in detail and incorporated the information as much as I can. Some sections of the handbook have been expanded and altered but, as there have been no major advances in understanding the causes of salicylate sensitivity or in its management and treatment, the core information remains the same.

Over the years, I have experimented with my diet a great deal and I have incorporated the useful aspects of those experiments in this new edition. I am still salicylate sensitive but things have become easier over the years.

I sincerely hope you find the information in this handbook useful and I wish you every success in finding a path to a truly wonderful state of health.

My very best wishes,
Sharla

Essential Information

The Salicylate Handbook has been written to provide information on the ways in which a salicylate sensitivity can affect the health of some individuals.

It is not my intention, nor should it be seen as being my intention, to provide medical advice or diagnosis. I am a researcher and writer, NOT a doctor.

As there are many possible causes of illness, it is essential that at all times you consult with your doctor or other medical practitioner. Any proposed changes to your diet should be discussed with your doctor or other medical practitioner before being started.

Under absolutely NO circumstances should you stop taking prescribed medication without the consent of your doctor.

It is my hope that you will find the information in this book useful and helpful but the responsibility for what you do with the information you read is completely your own. Please look after yourself really well.

Sharla Race

1 Salicylate Sensitivity

Just what is salicylate?

Well, the word "salicylate" is derived from the botanical name for the willow family which is "salicaceae". As far back as the first century, bark from the white willow was used to help relieve pain and inflammation but it wasn't until the early 1800s that the active ingredient was identified as being "salicin" and was later termed "salicylic acid". Then in 1838 salicylic acid was isolated from willow bark and, by 1899, acetylsalicylic acid was synthesised and marketed as "Aspirin".

We come into contact with salicylate in two forms:

1. In its natural form in vegetables, fruit, herbs, spices, and other plants.
2. Manufactured salicylate in products such as medicines, solvents, flavourings and perfumes.

Natural Salicylate

In plants, salicylate appears to exist as a naturally occurring preservative or insecticide protecting the plant and elongating its life span. The terms "sodium salicylate" and "salicylic acid" are often used to refer to this type of salicylate.

Salicylate is one of a multitude of chemicals that occur naturally in food. Virtually every meal we ever eat contains some salicylate and for most people this causes no problem but for an individual who is salicylate sensitive the consequences for their long-term health, if not diagnosed, can be disastrous. Wood et al identified the primary sources of salicylates in our diets as coming from alcoholic drink, herbs and spices, fruit and fruit juices, tomato based sauces, and vegetables (in that order).[1]

Natural forms of salicylate also find their way into many non-food products. For example, you will find methyl salicylate (oil of wintergreen) in many over the counter ointments, lotions and oils prescribed for muscle and joint pains as well as in other medicines and products such as mouthwashes and toothpastes. Oil of wintergreen contains 98% methyl salicylate and ingestion of 5ml of oil (about 1 teaspoon) is equivalent to 700 mg of aspirin—a dose that could be fatal to a young child.[2]

Man Made Salicylate

Salicylic acid, also known as "ortho-hydroxybenzoic acid", and other form of salicylate are used in the manufacture of various products including fungicides, resins, adhesives, dyes and medicines.

Salicylic acid is usually produced from phenol (carbolic acid). It was first synthesised and manufactured from phenol by Kolbe and Lautemann in 1860. The most commonly known form of man-made salicylate is "acetylsalicylic acid", what we know as "Aspirin".

There are also further groupings of chemicals that are not salicylate as such but are so similar in chemical structure that they can cause problems for those with a salicylate sensitivity. These include food additives such as the antioxidants BHA, BHT and TBHQ, and colours such as tartrazine. Throughout this handbook I refer to these type of substances as "salicylate mimics".

Aspirin (Acetylsalicylic acid)

Feinman, a toxicologist and microbiologist, writes that new benefits from aspirin use are being announced frequently: "At the same time, however, aspirin use can inadvertently cause illness and death for some individuals".[3]

Aspirin is used in the treatment of a wide range of conditions including muscle and joint pain, high temperatures and fevers, headaches, and in the prevention of heart disease. It is readily absorbed from the stomach and upper small intestine and once in the blood stream it is converted to salicylic acid.

Some people who are sensitive to aspirin have no problem with salicylate in food but individuals who have a sensitivity to salicylate in food invariably react also to aspirin. This is because salicylate, regardless of the type that it is, will, if the elimination process is not adequate or if large amounts are ingested, accumulate within the body. How soon reactions take place will depend on the individual's tolerance level.

A study of aspirin allergy by Speer et al in 1981 found that 90% of those with aspirin sensitivity were also sensitive to inhalants, food or other drugs.[4] Others, including Thune and Granholt,[5] and Park et al,[6] had similar findings. A study in 2000 by George et al found that many aspirin sensitive individuals also had adverse reactions to foods that contain natural salicylate.[7]

Eriksson's research found a high incidence of food sensitivity in acetylsalicylic acid-intolerant individuals that was probably explained by additives in foods as well as salicylates or benzoates naturally occurring in some food.[8]

The development of aspirin and its frequent use have provided us with a great deal of information on potential adverse reactions and how to deal with them. I will be using some of this information later in this handbook.

Salicylate Intolerance

If an individual is sensitive to salicylate, unwanted symptoms will appear when the level of salicylate in the body reaches a certain point. The point at which salicylate causes problems varies from individual to individual. If the amount of salicylate is reduced, the symptoms usually abate. Because of this, the symptoms are unlikely to be present all the time.

This section deals with symptoms, diagnosis, testing, causes and treatment. A summary of the key points follows:

- The degree of sensitivity varies enormously but most people, when they first discover they are salicylate sensitive, find they can tolerate very little ingested salicylate.
- Some people will react to all forms of salicylate whether ingested, inhaled or applied. Others will only react to one or two types and some react only to the larger doses found in medicines. Not everyone with a salicylate sensitivity reacts severely to inhaled salicylate.
- Age affects the severity of the sensitivity. The older you are when you discover the problem the longer it seems to take to "settle" the system and the degree of sensitivity tends to be more extreme.
- The sensitivity may diminish over time but for some individuals will always exist.
- Salicylate sensitivity may be an inherited condition in some cases but research also shows that in some cases it is not.
- The cause of salicylate sensitivity is not known although various theories have been put forward.

- Salicylate sensitivity is not an allergy and conventional testing methods are of little helping in diagnosing the condition.
- The main form of "treatment" is avoidance/reduction.

Symptoms

Adverse reactions to salicylate have been noted over the years—back in 1901, Dr. J. Dixon Mann developed stomach problems and decided to test a bottle of his usual cider drink. He found that it was high in salicylic acid and put forward the view that the salicylic acid was the cause of his stomach problems. He wasn't believed—at the time there was great interest in the use of salicylic acid as a preservative in food canning so there was always a backlash against anyone saying that salicylic acid caused problems.[9]

Salicylate intolerance, for some, can lead to a bewildering array of symptoms. The brain is often seriously affected as an overdose of salicylate first stimulates and then depresses the central nervous system leading to emotional and behavioural problems as well as physical problems. Over use of methyl salicylate (oil of wintergreen) can lead to salicylate poisoning in individuals who are not salicylate intolerant.[10]

Many of the symptoms that arise as a result of salicylate intolerance mimic those of allergy but a reaction to salicylate is not an allergy. Salicylate is cumulative in the body and symptoms will only arise when the tolerance level of the individual has been exceeded. The point at which symptoms arise is very individual specific and is also affected by various factors including age, weight, and general health.

A large number of symptoms and conditions have been linked with salicylate sensitivity and these are outlined in the lists below. The symptoms are unlikely to all appear at the same time in any one individual and for some salicylate sensitives only one or a few of the symptoms arise when their tolerance level is exceeded. Evidence from research on some of these conditions/symptoms can be found in Chapter 6.

Please note that anaphylactic reactions to aspirin have been recorded.[11] As far as I know there are no recorded instances of anaphylaxis to salicylate in food but extreme caution must be used when testing for a salicylate sensitivity. Lower doses of aspirin can give rise to mild salicylate intoxication with symptoms as varied as dizziness, tinnitus, diminished hearing and vision, headache, mental confusion, gastrointestinal problems, migraine, peptic ulcers/gastritis, depression, anxiety, psychiatric disorders, muscle and joint pain, pancreatitis, lassitude, drowsiness, sweating, thirst and breathing problems.[12]

When the level of salicylate reaches an extreme point, whether by accidental or intentional poisoning, then further symptoms are likely to develop. These can include anaemia, bleeding, coma, convulsions, EEG changes, haemorrhage, kidney problems, liver dysfunction, pulmonary oedema, and tachycardia.[13] If the salicylate levels are not reduced within the body then death can occur. Aspirin is not a drug to be taken lightly. There are some who doubt that if aspirin had been invented today that it would have been passed for everyday use let alone seen as a safe treatment for a whole host of conditions.

Although the amount of salicylate that is ingested from food is much lower, for some people it is still too much for their systems to deal with.

One of the aspects of a salicylate sensitivity that people newly diagnosed often find bewildering is that it seemingly arrives from nowhere. This is rarely the case. You can, if you look back, either notice symptoms that have recurred or identify a specific course of treatment from which time the problems stemmed.

Identified Salicylate Symptoms: Mainly Physical

Abdominal pain
Aching legs
Asthma
Bed wetting
Bladder Problems
Dermatitis
Dizziness
Ear Infections
Eye muscle disorders
Fatigue
Headaches
Hives
Hypoglycaemia
Nasal polyps
Persistent cough

Physical sluggishness
Poor physical co-ordination
Psoriasis
Reading/Writing problems
Rhinitis
Sinusitis
Sleep disorders
Skin problems
Speech difficulties
Stomach irritation
Swelling of face, hands, feet
Tics
Tinnitus
Urticaria
Visual Problems

Identified Salicylate Symptoms: Emotions, Behaviour and Feelings

Accident proneness
Anxiety and agitation (no reason)
Bouts of excessive energy followed by fatigue
Confused thinking
Depression
Distraction
Dyslexia
Excessive or constant talking
Hyperactivity
Impatience
Lack or loss of concentration

Memory problems
Mental sluggishness
Mood swings
Needing to be left alone
Nervousness
Sudden bouts of paranoia
Suicidal thoughts
Poor self image
Sudden highs
Temper flare ups
Unpredictability
Workaholism

For those who appear to have always had a salicylate sensitivity the point of breakdown, i.e. that time when your body can simply not continue and makes you very ill, is not predictable. Each of us has a unique biochemical makeup which will affect when this takes place. I will try explain this, and the more general process, a little more by using myself as an example.

1. For whatever reason, my body has never been able to deal with salicylate in any form except in small amounts.

2. Over the years, it did the best it could to help keep me going. The recurring symptoms and bouts of illness were all warnings that there was a problem but the cause was never diagnosed.

3. The various symptoms (such as rashes, joint pain, and overwhelming tiredness) did not respond to any form of treatment and all tests were negative. The symptoms always abated. There is no mystery to this, it is very simple—the body had managed to eliminate the excess salicylate and once the level was lowered the symptoms abated. Cyclical bouts of illness or behavioural patterns are extremely common amongst those who are salicylate sensitive but have not yet been diagnosed.

4. In my thirties, my health totally collapsed. This happened at a time when I had experienced a number of major changes in my life—job, area I lived in, house, marriage. The factor that seemed to act as the final trigger was a further job change which involved spending long lengths of time away from home in strange environments and eating only restaurant food. My

system quite simply had had enough and was tipped from "still managing" mode to "not coping".

5. The health collapse was a more serious warning that there was a problem that needed treating. My doctor continued to believe that there was nothing wrong with me (except for stress). More usually, at this point people are often sent for tests and investigations in hospital, the results of which are usually all negative.

6. This time, resting did not achieve anything. My body had now reached a point from which it could not recover without the appropriate help.

7. Reducing my dietary salicylate level to virtually zero was the treatment it needed. Within days, recovery began to take place.

8. After a period of time of being used to having little salicylate in my diet my tolerance level was reduced and I began to react to salicylate in products that were inhaled with the same symptoms (and a few new ones!).

9. However, the inhaled reactions were not in fact a new problem. They had always been present but simply not recognised before. When I thought back over the years I was able to see signs of this. For example, supermarket aisles with detergents always made me cough, I avoided wearing most perfumes, I disliked air fresheners and highly scented products and so on.

10. Reducing the number of inhaled sources of salicylate led to a reduction of the symptoms.

11. Maintaining a low salicylate diet and salicylate free environment helped my body recover.

12. As my body now has only low levels of salicylate, except after accidental exposure, I can tolerate larger amounts as long as these are not too frequent.

Diagnosis

Given the range of symptoms outlined above and the evidence presented in Chapter 6 you could be thinking that surely if all that information is available then doctors would have identified salicylate sensitivity as a possible cause of your problems. Unless you are fortunate to have a doctor who knows about salicylate sensitivity then this is unlikely to have happened for the following reasons:

- Salicylate sensitivity is not an accepted condition especially when it is not directly related to aspirin.

- Even when the sensitivity has arisen as a result of aspirin, or some other medication, it is not always diagnosed as such. For example, in hospitals, cases of salicylate poisoning are not always diagnosed correctly especially if the patient is older and the salicylate intoxication has been accidental.[14] Twenty seven per cent of patients hospitalised with salicylate intoxication, in a study by Anderson et al, were undiagnosed for as long as 72 hours after admission.[15] This delay in treatment inevitably led to deaths that could have been prevented with an earlier diagnosis. What chance does your ordinary doctor have if you present with less serious symptoms?

- The symptoms of salicylate sensitivity are many, confusing in their presentation, and often very individual specific.

- There is no recognised protocol for identifying the condition.

- If no medication is involved then the doctor has no objective indicator that points to salicylate as the problem. Salicylate sensitivity manifests at different times of life for different people. For some, with hindsight, it can be seen to have always been present but for others some event like prolonged use of aspirin or a similar drug can trigger the sensitivity.

Looking back over my own symptoms it is hard to criticise the medical profession for not identifying the true nature of my problems. Why would they have made the connection between my eye problems (nystagmus), fluctuating weight, strange aches and pains, accident proneness and lack of co-ordination as a child with salicylate?

What about the constant sinusitis, muscle and joint pain, tinnitus, skin rashes, the feelings of disassociation and strange mood swings, memory loss, the hyperactivity of workaholism followed by bouts of illness usually put down to viruses? The emergency room admission with severe back pain put down to a kidney infection that was never identified? The ear pain that nearly sent me crazy? The swollen abdomen, the continuing weight fluctuations?

Well once again no doctor ever saw all of these in one go but I suspect even if they had no link would have been made to salicylate. My experience of western doctors is very much that there is rarely a search for a cause. I was mystified when the hospital diagnosed me as having a kidney infection yet the tests were all negative. The pain during that time was so acute that I could walk less than a few steps. Eventually, after they sent me to be tested for a variety of tropical diseases (I had travelled abroad in the preceding few months) and all those tests also came back negative I was simply told to rest and yes it did eventually pass but neither they nor I were any the wiser.

I am sure this episode was caused by a diet change whilst abroad that included far more salicylate than I had ever eaten before and for a protracted length of time. Kidney problems and salicylate are not unknown.[16] A diagnosis of salicylate sensitivity could have saved me more than twenty years of misery but the one question that might have pointed us in the right direction was never asked—that question was "have you recently experienced any changes to your diet?"

Years later, I was told by one doctor that I must have developed post viral syndrome but that she didn't believe in the condition (not the most helpful of souls). No indication was made of what virus I may have had in the first place. I don't remember having one as such but I did have a bewildering array of symptoms including muscle and joint pain, no energy, angioedema and very pale blotchy skin, my hair was lifeless and my whole zest for life had vanished. Again the treatment was to rest and yes eventually I recovered but once again I was none the wiser.

Another time, my joint pain became so bad in one knee that any pressure was excruciating. My doctor said "arthritis" I asked why, the doctor said "why should you be any different" and told me to lose weight. In my bones, pun intended, I knew it wasn't arthritis and insisted on x-rays and yes they showed a totally clear joint. Did this help in a search for causes? On the contrary it was now decided that muscle strengthening exercises would help and I was sent away. I could see that the doctor now doubted the very existence of the pain.

Sadly, I could continue for pages with many more examples but I shall stop there. What I am trying to show is that when we present symptoms in isolation from each other it is virtually impossible for a doctor to make a diagnosis of salicylate sensitivity—there simply are not sufficient clues. In many ways only you will be able to see the connection.

It is also the case that as adults we will have come to accept many of the behavioural problems as simply being part of who we are. Either that or waste a lot of money and time on therapy of one sort or another. If we had presented with any of the "mental" symptoms we are likely to have been told we were under stress or been given medication for a psychological disorder. It is highly unlikely that our diet and environment would have been examined for any clues as to the cause of our problems.

Salicylate sensitivity is a hidden problem for many and until doctors accept its reality many children and adults will continue to suffer unnecessarily. As Dr Shelley writes: "The sophistication of modern medicine leads us to look for more and more complex causes of disease. Molecular biology, genetic drift, and spin resonance become our concepts. And yet... the following case illustrates how the obvious and the simple can cause a strange rare disease."[17] The case in question is described in some detail below and very clearly demonstrates that often the answer lies in what we eat and the plants and chemicals we come into contact with rather than some mystery illness that requires tests and treatments that never seem to resolve the underlying problem.

The case in question was of a six-year-old boy with generalised pustular psoriasis (psoriasis characterised by pus-like blisters on the skin usually on the hands or feet) due to a sensitivity to salicylates found in trees, shrubs, and medicines. It very clearly illustrates how a diagnosis of salicylate sensitivity can be difficult to arrive at, yet once arrived at seems obvious.

In April 1961 the child's condition was diagnosed as "generalized pustular psoriasis". The cause, despite extensive hospital tests, was unknown. The condition spontaneously cleared up but the child was then readmitted to the hospital in April 1964 with the same condition affecting over 80% of his body. The eruptions were accompanied by a high temperature. Hospital treatment was with a variety of drugs including aspirin. The pustular psoriasis continued to spread until all of his body was covered and his condition began to deteriorate.

Thankfully, investigations showed a sensitivity to aspirin and once this was removed from his treatment the condition began to improve and the boy went on to make a full recovery.

Once the critical factor of aspirin sensitivity had been identified, the pieces of the diagnostic puzzle fell into place. As aspirin sensitivity is a salicylate sensitivity, a search was made for previous salicylate exposure. Both attacks that had led to hospitalisation had taken place at the same time of the year and only in the years when he was living in the mountains of eastern Pennsylvania. The time of the year indicated that pollen may be a problem and it was found that sweet birch was common and that pollen from the catkins was very prevalent in early April.

It was then discovered that the young boy spent a great deal of time in the woods and was given to chewing birch leaves and twigs, and teaberry leaves (all very high in natural salicylate).

Interestingly, further investigations showed that the parents were able to remember times when less serious skin eruptions had appeared after the boy had chewed teaberry leaves. It was also found that other family members experienced some reactions to aspirin; his mother had a flushed reaction and an aunt developed psoriasis after using aspirin. The doctors concluded that the child was salicylate sensitive and needed to avoid it in all its form—natural and man made. By the way, the first hospital stay was much shorter because only a single aspirin dose had been administered and hence the condition had not been prolonged and exacerbated as it was during the second stay.

If you carry out your own research into salicylate sensitivity you will soon discover studies that question the existence of the condition. For example, Janssen et al argue that salicylates in food are unlikely to affect behaviour because, they believe, the level in food is too small.[18] My views on these type of studies are simple—ignore them. If that seems harsh it is meant to be. Since I started the *food can make you ill* web site web site, I have been moved and angered by many stories where serious problems have turned out to be caused by foods and food chemicals and far too often little, if any, help has been forthcoming from the medical profession. If you establish or suspect that you, or your child, has a food intolerance problem don't doubt it, deal with it. I hope you can take your doctor with you but if not rest assured you are far from being alone.

So, how do you know if you are salicylate sensitive?

Check the symptom lists. How many of the symptoms do you currently have or have frequently had before? The greater the number the more likely you are to be sensitive. Have you had periods of times when you have experienced clusters of the symptoms? Clustering and periodic bouts of symptoms are very common.

Salicylate sensitivity is generally a life-long condition and a pattern of symptoms and behaviour will usually be noticeable. Do you have an aversion to, or have felt very ill after eating, spices, herbs, fruit or vegetables? This is not necessarily an indicator as we have often been conditioned about our responses but think back to childhood and how you responded to these at that time.

Some believe that a salicylate sensitivity is an inherited condition. If, from the above, questions, you feel that you are probably salicylate sensitive you may be able to identify similar traits in another family member. Some caution is needed here—the extent of the sensitivity will vary and salicylate sensitive people often find ways of coping that mask their problem so it may not be immediately obvious and they may not be open to you suggesting that they have a salicylate sensitivity.

If there is no noticeable pattern but you are aware of a time when you were using a salicylate-based drug for a continuous period of time think back to how you were before this treatment. It would appear that for some individuals the condition is triggered by prolonged use of salicylate drugs.

Testing

Various tests exist to ascertain a sensitivity to aspirin and other drugs, and your doctor can arrange these types of tests but there "are no effective diagnostic tests for salicylate intolerance"[19]. Tests to establish a sensitivity to salicylate in food are much harder to come by as there is no agreed method of testing in use.

Please do not be misled by testing services that claim they can identify a salicylate sensitivity—check with your doctor before taking any of these. In some hospitals and allergy clinics a provocation test is administered to see if there is an adverse reaction—this is often carried out after a low salicylate diet has been followed for a period of time.

The administration of a provocation test is far more for the doctor's benefit than for the individual being tested—it provides the doctor with an objective method of saying yes this individual has a sensitivity to salicylate. The individual, him or herself, may not feel the need to have the provocation test as a low salicylate diet can, for many people who are salicylate sensitive, bring about major improvements in their symptoms within two to seven days. Skypala suggests that avoiding foods that are high in salicylate is sufficient enough a test if done over a four week period. She suggests that the reduction in salicylate will be enough to reduce symptoms and hence indicate whether the diet needs to be even lower in salicylate.[20]

The reason an improvement can be noticed so quickly has to do with the fact the body has suddenly been given a chance to eliminate the excess salicylate and quite simply does that. As the salicylate level is reduced, the symptoms just fade away. It is quite amazing when you experience this happening.

Once it has been decided that an individual is salicylate sensitive, the challenge is then to establish just how much dietary salicylate can be tolerated and a doctor is not able to do this except by providing a diet that is low in salicylate— this stage of the process will always involve trial and error.

The protocol described below relates primarily to salicylates in food and is based on my own experience. The easiest way to determine if you are salicylate sensitive is to reduce the level of salicylate in your system and the only way of doing this is to eat food containing no salicylate or very low levels, and to avoid salicylate in toothpastes, mouthwashes, herbal remedies and medications. Once the body has eliminated the stored salicylate, it is then possible to reintroduce foods containing a higher level and to assess the extent of any reaction.

If you suspect that salicylates may be a problem for you and you are taking any medication containing aspirin or another form of salicylate DO NOT undertake this test.

Check ALL your prescribed and over the counter medicines first. If in doubt, ask your doctor and/or pharmacist. Ideally, all medications should also be additive (especially colour) free. If you are taking a salicylate medication then consult your doctor before even considering this test. Please do take the above advice seriously. Aspirin, and other salicylate-based drugs, contain a very concentrated form of salicylate. If you stop taking them, reduce the overall salicylate level in your system, and then take one you could be putting your life at risk—death can result from anaphylactic shock.

As to how much salicylate each of us consumes depends very much on our diet. The estimated daily intakes have ranged from 0.4 to 200mg/day.[21] The points below may help give these figures some meaning.

1. Challenge testing has been carried out with a 300mg aspirin tablet.
2. The usual adult dose of aspirin is two 300mg tablets.
3. Asthma has been triggered in aspirin sensitives at doses between 45mg and 325mg .[22]

Under no circumstances attempt a challenge test at home using aspirin or any other form of salicylate—you could do yourself serious harm. If you want to undergo a challenge test discuss the option with your doctor, allergist or other healthcare provider.

Please do no think that a challenge test is an easy option. You would still have to follow a low salicylate diet for a period of time before a challenge test can be administered. This is essential because salicylate is cumulative in the body and you need to substantially lower the level prior to any form of testing—if you don't do this the results will not be clear. Do check the length of time you will be monitored for after a provocation test—Raithel et al note that whilst acute symptoms may only take a few hours to develop, chronic symptoms such as abdominal pain and skin itching may not appear until a few days later.[23]

A challenge test will then only tell you if you are sensitive to salicylate, it will not determine at what level the problem occurs. This can only be done by gradually increasing the number of salicylate foods in the diet until unwanted symptoms appear and then making the relevant adjustments and this can only be carried out after the overall salicylate level in the body has been reduced.

My own preference is for using the low salicylate diet outlined below and using the degree of symptom improvement as an indicator as to whether salicylate is a problem or not. It does seem to be the case that, if you are salicylate sensitive, then reducing the level in the diet brings improvements in symptoms within days and, for me, that is evidence enough. If your health practitioner has you removing other food chemicals or foods at the same time as reducing salicylate then you will probably need the provocation test as it will be difficult to determine which food or food chemical was causing the problems.

Because of the cross reactivity with certain additives and salicylate you would be wisest to avoid as many additives as possible during this testing period. Ideally you would try a diet for two weeks that was additive free and then move onto a low salicylate diet.

Low Salicylate Diet

As salicylate is cumulative in the body, you need to lower your level over a period of at least two weeks. During this time, you must be absolutely certain that you do not expose yourself to any high levels. Choose your fortnight with care as meals away from home will be very difficult to deal with. Food lists are given below and include numbers for scoring which may help you.

You can eat any amount of the foods listed as safe. If you are currently a vegetarian do not suddenly start eating meat, if you know that lettuce or one of the other foods makes you ill or you have an aversion to it then don't eat it—stick to foods you are used to eating, you can (if you want to) try the other ones later. Please ensure that you avoid all suspect food additives (see the section on Food Additives in Chapter 2).

To make it easier for you the categories of foods have been allocated a number so that you can keep score of how much salicylate you are eating—the score relates to an average portion. Your maximum allowance during this fortnight is FIVE a day and it is essential that you do not exceed this amount on any day. Keep a food diary and write down the total score for each day. Your food diary is going to become an incredibly important ally in unravelling your food sensitivities. Use it fully.

None of us are perfect and if you slip up don't beat yourself up about it. Correct it. If you find that on one day you unwittingly had a score of ten then make sure the next day's score is zero. Do not do the reverse—this means that if, for example, on the Friday, you scored three you must not increase Saturday's score to seven. KEEP TO FIVE. If you have slipped up on more than two consecutive days you may need to start your fortnight again.

At the end of the fortnight you will need to decide on the next stage. The degree of your sensitivity, your age, your overall health and the speed at which your body can detoxify will all have influenced what took place. You will probably find yourself in one of the following categories:

There was no noticeable change

If you had no improvement in your symptoms then it is unlikely that you are salicylate sensitive. You can test this by eating as many foods from the high lists as you like. If after a fortnight these cause you no problem you can safely assume that you do not have a problem with salicylates.

There was a gradual improvement in symptoms

If there was a gradual improvement then you are probably salicylate sensitive. It may be worth continuing with the very low salicylate diet for a further fortnight before trying to increase your salicylate level gradually. Then, increase your score allowance to ten a day over a two-week period. If your symptoms begin to get worse again drop your level to five for a few days and then increase slowly until you find the level you can tolerate.

If you can tolerate a score of ten a day then increase to fifteen a day, once again for two weeks, and keep on doing this until you reach the level at which your symptoms reappear. The easiest way of dealing with a return of symptoms is drop your level to five for a few days and then take it back up when you feel better.

There was no change at first then...

you had two or three days of feeling wonderful followed by days of being generally unwell and very tired—not too dissimilar to flu symptoms. This is detoxification and nothing to be unduly concerned about.

If you had a few days of feeling great and then feeling generally ill and tired it is likely that you have some degree of salicylate sensitivity. To give your body a chance to detoxify it is safest if you stay at this level for at least a further two weeks.

There was a substantial improvement in symptoms

A substantial improvement in symptoms indicates a salicylate sensitivity. You can try to gradually increase the amount of salicylate in your diet (using the scoring system) but the moment that you experience symptoms reduce the level for a few days. You may find that you can only eat foods from the categories below moderate (this is not unusual).

If you experience a reaction, be gentle with yourself. If salicylates affect your mind you may find it useful, when well, to write yourself a note you can read when a reaction takes hold—it should explain what is happening and reassure you that it will pass. If you have someone who understands what is happening talk to them—sometimes this helps minimise the anxiety.

If you have a child who experiences these problems it is essential that you reassure them that the symptoms will pass and that they are okay. Ensure that they are safe—you may need to limit the type of activities they are involved with during these times not so much by stopping them but by protecting them from involvement if they do not feel able to participate. Some children will be able to articulate their feelings whilst others will become withdrawn—they will be experiencing confusion, uncertainty and will feel lost, and frightened.

Increase the number of safe fruit and vegetables you can eat as this increases the alkalinity of your blood and helps your body eliminate salicylate. If your blood sugar has been affected, don't worry. Eat lots of small meals for as long as you need. If you need to rest then take the time do so. It will pass. The length and severity of reactions will vary from individual to individual but, as it takes time for the body to eliminate salicylate, you can expect to experience symptoms for at least a few days.

Please familiarise yourself with the all sections of this handbook before embarking on a long-term low salicylate diet and do please check with your doctor first.

Establishing a salicylate tolerance level is not an easy process and it can lead to a restrictive diet which is why many doctors advice against it. Depending on your age and other factors unique to you, you may find that over a period of time you will be able to tolerate more salicylate. I suspect that at first, for some of us, our bodies are so relieved to have a reduction in the toxin that they rebel at the input of any but when the body has had time to recover it is usually more able to deal with eliminating salicylate and hence able to accept more.

References

[1] Wood A, Baxter G, Thies F, Kyle J, Duthie G. A systematic review of salicylates in foods: estimated daily intake of a Scottish population. Mol Nutr Food Res. 2011 May;55 Suppl 1:S7-S14.

[2] DasGupta, A. Effects of Herbal Supplements on Clinical Laboratory Test Results (Patient Safety). Walter de Gruyter & Co, 2011.

[3] Feinman S (ed). Beneficial and Toxic Effects of Aspirin. CRC Press 1994.

[4] Speer F. Aspirin allergy: a clinical study. South Med J 1975;68(3):314-8.

[5] Thune P, Granholt A. Provocation tests with antiphologistica and food additives in recurrent urticaria. Dermatogica 1975;151:360-64.

[6] Park HS et al. Sodium salicylate sensitivity in an asthmatic patient with aspirin sensitivity. J Korean Med Sci 1991;6(2):113-7.

[7] George R, Zacharisen M, Kelly K. Frequency of reactions to foods containing natural salicylates in aspirin sensitive patients. AAAAI 56th Annual Meeting 2000.

[8] Eriksson NE. A relationship between food sensitivity and birch pollen-allergy and between food sensitivity and acetylsalicylic acid intolerance. Allergy 1978;33(4):189-96.

[9] Duckwall, EW. Canning and Preserving of Food Products with Bacteriological Technique. Pittsburghgh printing company, 1905, p.232.

[10] Chan TY. Potential dangers from topical preparations containing methyl salicylate. Hum Exp Toxicol 1996;15(9):747-50.

[11] Flarup M, Udholm S. Tardive anaphylactic shock caused by intolerance to aspirin.. Ugeskr Laeger 1989;151(35):2211-2.

[12] Feinman S. Aspirin Toxicity in: Feinman S (ed). Beneficial and Toxic Effects of Aspirin. CRC Press 1994, 23-30.

[13] Ibid.

[14] Lemesh RA. Accidental chronic salicylate intoxication in an elderly patient: major morbidity despite early recognition. Vet Hum Toxicol 1993;35(1):34-6.

[15] Anderson RJ, Potts DE, Gabow PA, Rumack BH, Schrier RW. Unrecognized adult salicylate intoxication. Ann Intern Med 1976;85(6):745-8.

[16] D'Agati V. Does aspirin cause acute or chronic renal failure in experimental animals and in humans? Am J Kidney Dis 1996;28(1 Suppl 1):S24-9.

[17] Shelley WB. Birch Pollen and Aspirin Psoriasis: A Study in Salicylate Hypersensitivity. JAMA 196428;189:985-8.

[18] Janssen PL, Hollman PC, Reichman E, Venema DP, van Staveren WA, Katan MB. Urinary salicylate excretion in subjects eating a variety of diets shows that amounts of bioavailable salicylates in foods are low. Am J Clin Nutr. 1996 Nov;64(5):743-7.

[19] Skypala, I. 'Other Causes of Food Hypersensitivity' in 'Food hypersensitivity: diagnosing and managing food allergies and intolerance', Skypala, I (Ed),Venter, C (Ed), Wiley-Blackwell, 2009.

[20] Ibid.

[21] Wood A, Baxter G, Thies F, Kyle J, Duthie G. A systematic review of salicylates in foods: estimated daily intake of a Scottish population. Mol Nutr Food Res. 2011 May;55 Suppl 1:S7-S14.

[22] Pauls JD, Siomon RA, Daffern PJ, Stevenson DD. Lack of effect of the 5-lipoxygenase inhibitor zileuton in blocking oral aspirin challenges in aspirin-sensitive asthamtics. Ann Allergy, Asthma, Immunol 2000;85:40-45.

[23] Raithel M, Baenkler HW, Naegel A, Buchwald F, Schultis HW, Backhaus B, Kimpel S, Koch H, Mach K, Hahn EG, Konturek PC. Significance of salicylate intolerance in diseases of the lower gastrointestinal tract. J Physiol Pharmacol. 2005 Sep;56 Suppl 5:89-102.

2 Salicylate in Food

As far as we know, the first published estimate of salicylic acid content of food appeared in an anonymous letter in the Lancet in 1903. The writer estimated that salicylic acid was present in strawberries and other fruits at a concentration of "1/64th of a grain/two pounds of fruit".[1]

In a textbook on preserving food that appeared in 1905 there was much interest in the levels of naturally occurring salicylate and benzoic acid in fruit and vegetables. Duckwall notes that raspberries, currants and horseradish contain salicylic acid: also, "Cherries, plums, crab-apples, grapes, strawberries, apricots and peaches, contain salicylic acid in appreciable quantities". Salicylate was also recognised as being present in tomatoes, cauliflower and string beans.[2]

In the 1960s and 70s lists of foods containing salicylate were available[3,4] but tended only to include:

Almonds
Apples
Apricots
Blackberries
Cherries
Currants
Gooseberries
Grapes
Nectarines

Oranges
Peaches
Plums
Raspberries
Strawberries
Birch Beer
Teaberry
Wines

The work of Anne Swain[5] and others in Australia in the mid 1980s demonstrated the extent to which salicylate is present in food and it is their findings that form the basis of the majority of salicylate food lists in use today.

Since then various other studies, including one by Wood et al[6], have looked at salicylate levels in food. None have been as extensive, in respect of the number of foods tested, as the Swain study and, unfortunately, rather than extending the information we have available have somewhat confused the picture. As Scotter et al point out, data on the salicylate content of foods are not only sparse but also contradictory.[7] I am delighted that other researchers have begun looking into salicylate in food but for someone with a salicylate sensitivity, and for their doctors, the conflicting information that is beginning to emerge is difficult to deal with.

In summary, the studies have all identified salicylic acid in fruit, vegetables, herbs and spices with spices always having the highest concentrations.

Reviewing the information for this edition of the *Salicylate Handbook*, I was faced with a dilemma. Did I try incorporate some of the newer studies into the main food lists or did I leave the lists as they were? As the lists had worked in helping people reduce their salicylate levels, and in beginning to understand what amount they are able to tolerate, I only did some minor tweaking, and expanding of the categories.

I strongly recommend that if you are new to understanding salicylate sensitivity you start with the lists provided by your doctor or, if none have been made available to you, with the lists below. Once you are comfortable with understanding how much salicylate your body can tolerate you can then "tweak" your diet with more confidence. The lists are not the end of the story—salicylate content may vary from different crops and harvests, not all foods are listed, results have not been retested and, in the future, newer methods of analysis may be discovered. It is however, the clearest list you will find available and, if you follow the guidelines in the previous chapter on testing, you should soon have an idea of whether you are salicylate sensitive and be able to establish your level of tolerance.

The food lists given below have been developed mainly from the article *Salicylates in foods* by Anne Swain et al,[8] but information from some other studies including Wood et al[9] has also been included. At the end of the lists is a supplement, *Not the end of the story,* which provides further information on salicylate content in food from other sources, and my own and others experience.

Over the years I have discovered some anomalies between the lists I included in the first Salicylate Handbook and my own experience. I have experimented on myself many times— increasing my salicylate levels and trying different foods. As we are all different, I would have hesitated in sharing some of this information with you but I am increasingly finding that my "anomalies" are being confirmed by more recent studies. So, I have given details of many of these and I hope that the information will help you in adjusting your diet to take in a wider range of foods. But, if you are just starting out, please stick with the lists below until you have got used to eating a diet that is low in salicylate. Whenever I give myself a problem I immediately fall back on eating from only the safe and very low food lists.

Various studies have found cross reactivity between certain additives and salicylate and these are outlined in the section on *Food Additives.*

For the purposes of testing it would be advisable to treat foods not on the main lists as suspect. You can experiment with them at a later stage when you can clearly determine what is happening. The categories of food are safe, very low, low, moderate, high, very high, extremely high, and mega high.

To place the lists in some perspective you should know that most salicylate sensitives can only eat foods from the safe, very low, and low lists; some even have problems with the low list. Having said that, do please remember that everyone is different.

Food Lists

Individual foods have been allocated a score depending on how high they are in salicylate. The numbers range from 0 to 7 and the categories are as follows:

0 = Safe Foods

1 = Very Low

2 = Low

3 = Moderate

4 = High

5 = Very High

6 = Extremely High

7 = Mega High

Safe Foods: score = 0

Fruit: Pear (fresh and peeled).

Vegetables: Bamboo shoots, cabbage—green/white, celery, lettuce (iceberg), swede. Potatoes—old white variety and peeled.

Legumes (dried): Brown lentils, black-eye beans, brown beans, chick peas, green split peas, lima beans, mung beans, red lentils, soya beans. You may use canned beans but avoid any that have added ingredients.

Grains: Barley, millet, oats, rice, rye, wheat. To avoid additives and hidden preservatives, all bread, biscuits, cakes etc... should be home-made.

Seeds and nuts: Poppy seeds.

Sweeteners: Maple syrup, white sugar.

Meat, fish, poultry: Beef, chicken, eggs, lamb, oysters, pork, salmon (canned), tripe, tuna (canned). Do not eat any processed meat.

Herbs, spices and condiments: Malt vinegar, saffron, salt, soy sauce.

Oils and fats: Butter. Oils such as rapeseed, safflower, soya bean, and sunflower which are free from additives. Non dairy spreads that are additive free and use the oils mentioned above.

Dairy: Butter, mild cheeses that are free from preservatives and colours, milk, yoghurt— natural only but you can add your own fruit.

Misc: Carob powder, cocoa, arrowroot.

Beverages: Decaffeinated coffee, home made pear juice, milk, water. Milks made from oats, rice and soya as long as they have no added flavours or preservatives.

Very Low Salicylate Foods: score = 1

Fruit: Banana, green golden delicious apple (peeled), honeydew melon, paw paw, pomegranate, tamarillo.
Vegetables: Brussels sprouts, chives, choko, garlic, green peas(fresh), leek, red cabbage, shallot.
Legumes: Borlotti beans, mung bean sprouts, yellow split peas.
Grains: Buckwheat.
Nuts and seeds: Cashew nuts.
Herbs, spices and condiments: Fennel (dried), fresh parsley.
Sweeteners: Golden syrup.
Meat and fish: Liver, prawns, scallop.
Dairy: Some cheeses including blue vein, camembert, and mozzarella.
Beverages: Camomile tea, decaffeinated black tea.

Low Salicylate Foods: score = 2

Fruit: Fresh figs, mango, passion fruit, persimmon, plums (without the skin), red delicious apple (peeled), rhubarb.
Vegetables: Fresh asparagus, beetroot, cauliflower, green beans, onion, marrow, pimiento, potato (with peel), pumpkin, tomato, turnip. spinach (frozen), sweetcorn.
Seeds and nuts: Hazelnuts, pecan, sunflower seeds.
Herbs, spices and condiments: Fresh coriander leaves.
Beverages: Pear juice (shop bought).

Moderate Salicylate Foods: score = 3

Fruit: Apples (most varieties), kiwi fruit, loquat, pear with peel.

Vegetables: Asparagus (canned), aubergine (no peel), beetroot (canned), black olives, carrot, lettuces other than iceberg, mushrooms, sweetcorn (niblets), tomato juice.

Seeds and nuts: Desiccated coconut, peanut butter, sesame seeds, walnuts.

Sweeteners: Molasses.

Beverages: Coco cola, lemonades.

High Salicylate Foods: score = 4

Fruit: Lemon, lychee, morello cherries, nectarine, watermelon.

Vegetables: Parsnips, white and yellow sweet potato.

Grains: Maize meal.

Seeds and nuts: Brazil nuts, macadamia nuts, pine nuts, pistachio nuts.

Herbs, spices and condiments: Horseradish, tabasco sauce. The amount of salicylate may vary according to the brand so be cautious.

Oils and fats: Almond oil, corn oil, peanut oil, sesame oil, walnut oil.

Beverages: Rosehip tea.

Very High Salicylate Foods: score = 5

Fruit: Apples (granny smiths), figs (dried), grapefruit, mandarin, peach, tangelo.

Vegetables: Alfalfa, avocado, baby squash (fresh), broad beans, broccoli, green chilli peppers, okra (canned), spinach (fresh), tomatoes (canned), yellow chilli peppers.

Oils and fats: Coconut, olive, sesame, walnut.

Beverages: Coffee.

Extremely High Salicylate Foods: score = 6

Fruit: Cherries (fresh), grapes, mulberries, strawberries.

Vegetables: Aubergine (with peel), chicory, endive, courgette, cucumber (no peel), green peppers, radish, watercress.

Condiments: Chilli powder, white vinegar.

Misc: Vegetable and yeast extracts.

Mega High Salicylate Foods: score = 7

Fruit: Apricots, blackberry, blackcurrant, blueberry, boysenberry, canteloupe melon, cranberry, cherries (canned), currants, dates (fresh), loganberry, guava, orange, pineapple, prunes, raisin, raspberry, red currant, sultana, youngberry.

Vegetables: Gherkins, mushrooms(Champignon), olives (green), red chilli pepper, water chestnut.

Nuts and seeds: Almonds, peanuts (with skin).

Sweetners: Honey.

Herbs, spices and condiments: White vinegar, vanilla essence. Most herbs and spices (see below)

Beverages: Peppermint tea.

Herbs and Spices : Virtually all herbs and spices also come into the mega high category. The Swain[10] study tested a range of these and I have broken them down into three categories—please remember all are in the mega high category it is just that some are higher than others.

Lowest	Medium	Highest
Allspice	Aniseed	Curry Powder
Basil	Canella	Dill
Bay Leaf	Cayenne	Garam Masala
Caraway	Cinnamon	Mixed Herbs
Cardamom	Cumin	Oregano
Clove	Fenugreek	Paprika
Ginger (fresh)	Mace	Rosemary
Mint (fresh)	Mustard	Thyme
Nutmeg	Sage	Turmeric
Pepper	Tarragon	
Pimento		

Alcohol

Alcohol varies in amount. Given the difficulty in fully ascertaining the ingredients of alcoholic beverages, it is best to avoid drinking alcohol during the first two weeks. The following list can be only be treated as a very basic guide to levels. The safest course of action would be to introduce your favourite drink as a test.

Gin, whisky and vodka are probably safe.

Beer, brandy, cider, and sherry generally have a high salicylate content.

Liqueurs, port, rum, and wine are extremely high in salicylate

Not the end of the story

The above lists make an excellent starting point but they are not the end of the story. I know it is frustrating not to have a definitive list but sadly that isn't currently possible. Various studies have disagreed on the salicylate content of foods and it is not possible to easily amalgamate them or compare them for the following reasons:

1. They used different varieties of fruit/vegetables.
2. The foods will have been grown in different ways (and in different countries).
3. We do not know if the foods had been treated in any way after being harvested.
4. The studies rarely use the same method of establishing salicylate content.

5. Not all studies provide information on what parts of a food were tested: for example, we often do not know if the peel/skin has been removed.

6. They rarely test the same foods.

It would be in fact be impossible to test all varieties of fruit, vegetables, herbs and spices and come up with any meaningful results. The amount of salicylate will always vary depending on the variety of the fruit, vegetable, herb or spice, and the way a crop has been grown, harvested, and stored. Variations in findings can at times be quite extreme. For example, in one study, the salicylate content of five brands of orange juice ranged from 0.47 to 3.01mg/L.[11]

During the early days of learning to live with a salicylate sensitivity, stick to the lists given above or to those provided by your doctor—if the ones provided by your doctor differ significantly from the lists in this book please always follow the lists from your doctor.

Eventually, you will want to do some experimenting but I would strongly advice that you do not do it until you are sure you understand how much salicylate you can get away with. You will also find it much easier if you use a food diary so that if a problem occurs you can identify the culprit more easily.

There are some anomalies that seem to pop up on regular basis regarding foods that salicylate sensitives have problems with including milk and wheat. I see a great deal of speculation as to what aspect of a food might be the culprit but the reality is that we don't know. It always strikes me that it is a sub set of salicylate sensitives that react to a range of foods that have generally been considered to be free from or very low in salicylate. Whilst I think discussion and sharing is important, it is also important not to get too sidetracked into having to understand every single little anomaly in the diet. Why? Because you are never going to get an answer to all the issues that come up. Sometimes you just have to accept that a food causes a problem and not worry about it. If you are a parent and have spotted that your child reacts to a supposedly salicylate free food then please trust yourself—it really doesn't matter what the lists tell you, if you have seen the change in behaviour and linked it with a specific food then eliminate the food.

It is amazing how complex each and every fruit, vegetable, spice and herb actually are: "It is important to be aware of the sheer numbers of plant bioactive compounds. Attention tends to be focused on a few representatives of each class, but 25,000 members of the terpenes have been identified, around 8000 phenolics and there are even 250 different sterols."[12] Lists can only ever serve as guidelines.

Alcohol

It is safest to avoid alcoholic drinks, like wine, sherry, and cider that are made from fruit. You may be able to tolerate some of the spirits mentioned in the food lists. Beers and lagers will vary enormously.

Assume nothing is safe and introduce your chosen drink as a test and monitor your reaction. I very rarely drink so the only option from my personal experience that I can offer as being free from, or very low in, salicylate is a Vodka made from peeled potatoes.

Be aware that low alcohol and alcohol free options can also be very high in salicylates—5-Hydroxysalicylic acid has been found in alcohol free beer.[13]

Alternative milks

Alternative milks such as oat, soya, and rice milk can pose a potential problem depending on how they have been manufactured. The commercial brands often contain additional ingredients such as apple juice, oils, and flavourings. Check the labels carefully. The packaging may also have been treated with additives.

If you use large amounts of these types of milks you might want to consider buying a soy milk machine which will enable you to make fresh milk whenever you need it and give you complete control of the ingredients. Soy milk machines can generally make milks using most grains such as rice and oats but check with the manufacturer before buying.

Breakfast Cereals

Cereals are low in salicylate but beware mass produced brands especially those with added vitamins as these vitamins have often been treated with antioxidants that can cause problems.

If you ever suspect a cereal is a problem do not assume that a new sensitivity has appeared—first test the suspect grain in its most natural form (mass produced breakfast cereals are not the way to do it). The chemicals used in processed food that do not have to appear on labels can be sources of hidden salicylate and misread as a new sensitivity that can lead to unnecessary diet restrictions.

See also the section on *Grains* below.

Cow's Milk

Salicylate levels in cow's milk are supposed to be negligible or non-existent yet cow's milk is a food that seems to cause problems for many salicylate sensitives.

The problems could result from contamination during the heating, transit, storage and packaging processes—residues from cleaning chemicals could conceivably be present in the final product and unfortunately this would apply to organic milk as well as "normal" milk.

I wonder if the problem is one that arises from packaging material. Could some additive or other chemical that is a salicylate mimic being leeched into the milk?

Some forms of milk, in some countries, have added vitamin A. So do check that you are buying milk that is just "milk". Food additives of various types, including antioxidants such as BHA and BHT, could conceivably have been used during various treatments in the manufacturing process. It is also possible that residues from some cattle treatments such as growth hormones and antibiotics could have survived the heat treatment processes and be present in the milk. There has also been speculation that naturally occurring hormones and other chemicals within milk can cause an overload within the human body—this theory suggests that because these chemicals require detoxification there is build up of salicylate in the system.

More recently there has been a move towards distinguishing between two types of milk depending on the type of protein "beta-casein" they contain—either A1 or A2. The A2 type is said to be higher in naturally occurring Beta Carotene (vitamin A), and Omega 3, and the Beta Casein A2 is said to be better tolerated by many people. The majority of milk that is readily available is A1. In the UK the main source of A2 comes from Guernsey herds.

My own experience with milk and milk products has been very mixed. I think I have tried pretty much most variations (except A2) and the one thing I am sure about is that milk is low in or free from salicylate. However, milk can and does cause many salicylate sensitives, myself included, problems and there appears to be no single reason that applies to everyone. As cows milk is often an important part of the diet, I suggest that you persevere and see if you can find an option that works for you.

In respect of butter, the ones I have had most success with have been from free range cows. Having said that, all forms of butter sooner or later make me bloat and some organic types have had me retching within minutes. I think the problem in some cases is simply that there are additives in the packaging or the added salt or there has been contamination somewhere along the way

In respect of cheese I have found that I can really only tolerate a very mild cheddar. I have found myself feeling exceedingly sick when I have tried cottage and cream cheeses.

Very few cheeses have been tested in respect of salicylate. The Swain study found the following levels:

Blue vein 0.05mg/100gm
Camembert 0.01mg/100gm
Cheddar 0.00
Cottage Cheese 0.0
Mozzarella 0.02mg/100gm

Be careful when buying cheese as some varieties/brands have added colourings.

If you can tolerate cow's milk then yoghurt will be a welcome addition to your diet. The natural type will always be safest and you can add your own fruit and sweeteners if you would like to. I have seen studies that have listed strawberry yoghurt as very low in salicylate[14] but unfortunately there is no mention as to whether the yoghurt contained real fruit or flavourings.

Chocolate

Cocoa is low in salicylate and so it is easy to make the assumption that all forms of chocolate are safe to eat. They are not. Beware of any flavoured chocolate whether it be with peppermint, strawberry, ginger or anything else. Your safest option is always going to be a plain chocolate bar—either milk or dark depending on whether you can tolerate milk or not.

The issue now becomes whether you can tolerate the vanilla or vanilla flavouring that has been added. Whilst it is generally thought that small amounts of vanilla essence are safe, all types of vanilla have not been tested and the range of options on the market today are numerous. My experience is that vanilla flavouring is never okay and that natural vanilla can also be a problem. One of the problems with real vanilla is to do with amount. If you only ever eat a very small amount of chocolate once in a while then the amount of vanilla (real vanilla) is unlikely to be a problem for you. However, if you eat chocolate every day or a few times in a week then the vanilla could become a problem.

So, what is the safest option? Most definitely a chocolate that has no vanilla added. These are not immediately easy to find but they do exist and what is available will depend on where you live. There is also the option of raw chocolate which can be made at home using the ingredients of your choice—search for "raw chocolate recipes" online and you'll find a number of options.

Flavourings and sauces

Yeast spreads, tomato sauces, gravy powders, brown sauces, tomato ketchups, stock cubes—all of these are most likely to be high in salicylate. The studies generally have them as high but some discrepancies do appear. For example, the Swain[15] study found 64.3mg/kg of salicylate in Worcestershire sauce whilst the Scotter[16] study found less than 0.2mg/kg.

If you really feel you can't live without them, check the ingredients lists and find the option that looks like it has the lowest amount of salicylate. When you try it, make sure you use a very small amount and monitor yourself carefully. It is worth periodically checking what's on the market as new products are continuously being introduced and the way existing products are manufactured is also regularly being changed.

At times I have had tiny (and I do mean tiny) amounts of yeast extract on a piece of toast. I have also at times used gravy powders. The danger of introducing some of these products into your diet is that you forget that they are high in salicylate and have a little too much or have them too regularly and then you suddenly find yourself feeling quite unhinged and unable to work out why. Whilst working on this new edition of the Salicylate Handbook that is exactly what I did and it wasn't a pleasant experience so my advice would be only use or make low salicylate versions.

Fruit

There have been discrepancies between studies on the salicylate content in fruit. Paterson et al outline these when they show that the Swain study had the following fruits as high or very high and the Janssen study as very low: apple, canned apricot, orange, strawberry, currants, and raisins.[17]

Reactions to raw fruit that are in theory low in salicylate are not unknown. For example, Breakey found that Golden Delicious apples with negligible amounts of salicylate were still not well tolerated.[18,19]

Don't give up on these fruits without trying them in different ways. My mouth can swell and I can develop mouth ulcers if I eat a golden delicious apple (peeled) when it is too green. Once the apples have yellowed I have no problem. I have also found that cooking the less ripe ones makes them totally safe for me. So experiment. The amount of salicylate in apples varies between varieties and some studies have them as very low[20], and others much higher[21].

As to limes well my own experiments with these have never resulted in a reaction so I suspect that they have substantially lower levels than lemons and a study in 2011 found them to be free of salicylate.[22] I use lime juice in drinks but would advocate against using lime peel in baking just in case of pesticide residues or salicylate.

I keep an organic lemon in the fridge and use a few drops of lemon juice in things like salads, tea, and homemade lemonade. I am cautious with lemon juice as I have sometimes experienced problems with it and at other times not. The Swain study found lemons to be low in salicylate but Scotter et al[23] found lemon to be the fruit with the highest amount but they found that drinks such as lemonade and bitter lemon to be very low in salicylate.

The Wood et al study found very low amounts of salicylate in grapes.[24] Other studies have generally found higher amounts in grapes. I have found that I can eat about five or six grapes (green or red) without any major problem but I don't keep them in my diet because I find it hard to limit myself to such a small amount and they are a fruit that is virtually impossible to peel. The red variety can brighten up a bland looking fruit salad—each grape can be sliced into between 6 and 8 pieces and when mixed in with peeled pear and honeydew melon gives the dish a good dose of colour.

The Scotter[25] study found that whilst green grapes had highish levels of salicylate, the levels in their dried versions, as currants and sultanas, was lower (a study by Venema found the opposite) and so they argue that salicylate is lost during the drying process. I am not keen on sultanas or raisins so can not comment on these but I can say that I do use small amounts of Vostizza currants when making cup cakes and have never experienced a problem with them.

The level of salicylate in strawberries and raspberries is usually seen as being high but the Wood et al study[26] found very low levels in raspberries. In respect of fruit, I tend to use the principle of *if you can't peel it, don't eat it* so I have no personal experience to offer here.

The Swain[27] study found the salicylate levels of oranges to be high whilst the Wood[28] and Scotter[29] studies found them to be low. I have tried oranges over the years and the only ones I can tolerate are the variety that are very large with a very thick skin. When I have a cold and want to increase my vitamin C levels I squeeze half of one of these oranges into water. I have done this for up to five days without experiencing any problems. I have also occasionally added pieces of this type of orange to fruit salads to add a bit of colour with no ill effects. I have had little success with smaller oranges and commercial orange juices are too concentrated for me.

The Scotter[30] study found clementines to be low in salicylate. No one appears to have tested satsumas—when they are in season, I occasionally eat half of one with no problem.

Nobody disputes that nectarines contain salicylate but some studies have them as being very high and others lower. I very nervously tried nectarines a few years ago and found them to be just fine and have gone on to enjoy them every summer since then. I only ever eat them peeled and rarely more than twice a week but they make a welcome change. Peaches which have been measured as having lower amounts of salicylate than nectarines have given me problems. I don't know if this is to do with the variety I tried, pesticides or some quirk of mine but the reaction I had was strong enough to dissuade from trying peaches again.

The amount of salicylate measured in plums seems to vary enormously. The Wood study found the level to be virtually zero (0.01mg/kg) and this finding fits with my own experience.

I have no problems with plums but I only eat them without their skins. Peeling plums is very messy but the flesh can be eaten out of the skins if you cut the fruit into quarters and twist it away from the stone. I have also eaten tiny amounts of plum jam that have been made with whole plums with no ill effects.

Traditionally, bananas have been classed as a safe food—free from salicylate. Some studies have found small amounts of salicylate in bananas; for example, Wood et al found 0.34mg/kg.[31] I have had problems with bananas over the years. The ones that cause me the least problems are small organic ones which leads me to wonder if the pesticides and fungicides used so widely in banana cultivation are the problem—it is quite conceivable that these contain salicylate and that the salicylate enters the edible part of the plant.

Fruit Juices

The concentrated nature of commercial fruit juices means they will always be high in salicylate. When the juice is made from whole fruits such as pear and apple, the juice will contain the salicylate that is present in the peel. It may also contain residues of any pesticides used.

Juice from fruits with harder peels such as orange, pineapple and pomegranate are made from the inner fruit so you are avoiding less pesticide contamination but many of these fruits are still high in salicylate.

Be aware that a large number of individual fruits go into producing a litre bottle of fruit juice so if the fruit is high in salicylate, the juice will be extremely high. To get a clearer idea of how much juice can be obtained from a single orange, squeeze one at home into a glass—commercial juicing machines will extract more but this experiment is about giving you a visual clue as to the amount of juice that is present in a single orange. If you really miss orange juice you could try half an orange squeezed into a glass and topped up with water (still or carbonated). I do this whenever I feel the need for a little extra vitamin C. Most times I have no problem with it but I have had instant stomach aggravation and a blood sugar dip and I can only assume that when this has happened I have managed to use an orange that was particularly high in salicylate. I'm afraid there is no way of definitely knowing which orange will be okay and which won't.

Pomegranates are thought to be fairly low in salicylate and I have drunk commercially squeezed pomegranate juice with no problems but I do add water and I would avoid it if my salicylate levels were high. Be cautious when buying pomegranate juice as it is a fruit that is frequently combined with other fruits.

You can make your own pear juice at home. Peel and dice some ripe pears, put them in a blender, add a little water, and blend until you have juice—add as much or as little water as you need. Blending pears with natural yoghurt also makes a very pleasant drink—it is also something that can be frozen as an ice lolly.

Grains

In theory grains are free from salicylate and most probably are but for some reason there appears to be a subset of salicylate sensitives, myself included, who react to many of them. What we know is that most of the plants whilst they are growing do contain salicylate whether it be in the root, leaves or shoots. Once the grain has been harvested the parts containing salicylate are usually discarded so the parts we eat are theoretically salicylate free.

So why do some salicylate sensitives react to wheat, buckwheat, even rice? I suspect the answer lies in the amount and type of phenolic acids in the grain. Salicylic acid itself is a phenol and some other phenols are very similar in respect of their chemical structure. The problem could also simply be a sensitivity to some other phenols. The phenolic content is always going to be the highest in outer part of the grain so unrefined grains will always be higher in their phenolic content[32,33.] This may explain why some salicylate sensitives can eat refined grains such as white rice and wheat but not their unrefined counterparts.

It is not going to be possible for me to give you a list of all the possible suspect phenols as there simply isn't one. My own guess is that the suspects are probably types of hydroxybenzoic acids: for example, one of these, vanillic acid, is found in rye grain,[34] oats,[35] brown rice,[36] refined wheat flour,[37] white rice,[38] white maize,[39] wheat bran,[40] parboiled rice[41].

Interestingly Dykes and Rooney identified sorghum and millet as having the widest variety of phenolic acids. They also, in their review, note that some studies have found salicylic acid in barley, sorghum, and wheat. The grains that had the lowest levels were white rice, dehulled barley, and white wheat.[42]

I have yet to meet a salicylate sensitive who does not have some degree of a problem with wheat. The Swain study found no detectable traces of salicylate in the grain but salicylate has been detected in wheat seed.[43] Basically I don't know if there is salicylate in wheat or not. I suggest that if you find you are having problems with it that you eliminate it from your diet, in all its forms, for at least five days and then try an organic white flour in something like a basic pancake mix. If you are okay with this then test it in a home made bread or biscuit. If you experience a reaction then it is some other ingredient like yeast that could be the problem.

If you find yourself okay with white flour then try a wholemeal flour and see if that is okay. It is important that you test various white flours, including organic ones, to try find one without a hidden ingredient that is a problem for you such as a bleaching agent (these are no longer allowed in the UK) or added nutrient like iron, thiamine, niacin or calcium carbonate which are compulsory in white flours in the UK. Please note that it is unlikely to be a nutrient that is the problem but it may be an additive used in manufacturing process. A while ago I was intent on finding a white flour I could use for making bread and kept trying various brands until I found one that caused the least problems—as companies change their suppliers of ingredients, I will change brands the moment I notice that I am not feeling quite right with the bread I make.

Yan et al report on two cases of anaphylaxis caused by dust mite infestation of wheat flour. In discussing their findings, they note that salicylate intolerance is often reported in individuals who have problems with mite infested foods.[44] Given this link it is probably wise to store flour, especially once it has been opened, in the fridge. Sánchez-Borges et al also found that there was a high prevalence of urticaria and angioedema reactions to aspirin and other nonsteroidal anti-inflammatory drugs in individuals who develop oral mite anaphylaxis.[45]

Whilst buckwheat is generally classed as being a safe food for those of us with a salicylate sensitivity it still appears to cause problems for many. The reason may be that the "hulled groats are about 0.7% phenolic compounds, some of which give the grain its characteristic astringency".[46] The distinctive aroma that buckwheat has, when heated, is caused by these and they include among their number salicylaldehyde

I have tried every variation of rice over the years and I now only use white basmati rice. Long and short grain rice (brown or white, as a grain or as a flour, organic/non-organic) messes with my blood sugar and gives me a coated tongue. I don't know why and this could just be a Sharla quirk so don't give it a second thought if you are just fine with the rice you are using.

The best piece of advice I can give is, if you think you are having a problem with a grain switch to a more refined version of it: for example, white wheat flour rather than whole-wheat, white rice rather than brown, light rye flour rather than dark. This just might work as the phenols are always more concentrated in the outer part of the grain.

Herbs

All the studies agree that salicylate levels in herbs are high. The only one that always scores low is parsley.

I have done very little experimenting with herbs as even the tiniest amounts of herbs such as basil or oregano were making me feel unwell. So, although I know the theory is that if you only use a little you should be okay I am unable to confirm it and would advocate against using herbs especially when they have been dried—they really are too concentrated. If you feel you have to use a herb then treat it as suspect and start with very, very small amounts.

Legumes (Pulses)

The majority of the legumes are classed as free from or very low in salicylate yet for some reason some of the legumes cause problems for some salicylate sensitives. The two most frequent culprits being soya and chick peas.

Soya causes many problems from severe anaphylaxis to minor stomach pains in a variety of people. The testing of the beans that has been done indicates that soy is free from salicylate and that is my own experience. However, I do find that I cannot eat processed soy as in flakes, minces or ready meals—I suspect that the processing has led to contamination with additives of some sort although it may also be something that is in the soy itself. I find that if I use soy milk (home made) for longer than a couple of weeks that I start to feel not quite right.

Interestingly, a paper by Süss et al presents the case of three individuals who experienced anaphylactic reactions to a soy drink. Cross-reactivity of soy protein with birch pollen allergens was identified as the cause for their severe reactions. The authors findings prompted them to write that anyone with a birch pollen allergy should avoid the intake of soy protein.[47] De Swert et al also found links between birch pollen allergy and soy allergy.[48] Raw soybean sprouts have also been found to contain gentisic acid which is an active metabolite of salicylic acid degradation.[49]

There are no similar findings as regards chick peas. I think we have to assume that there is something probably, in the outer skin, that is problematic for some salicylate sensitives. The reason I am betting on the outer skin is because if you look at the levels of salicylate in normal peas, the ones that have been split and had the skin removed are much lower in salicylate than their fresh from the pod cousins.

Not all legumes have been tested. The ones that I seem to be okay with are adzuki beans, brown lentils, cannellini beans, green lentils, haricot beans, and red kidney beans. I do not tolerate chick peas, red lentils or soya beans very well.

Nuts

The only nut that is low in salicylate is the cashew but some people, myself included, have reported problems with them. As the nutshell and other parts of cashew are quite high in salicylate[50] there could be contamination when the extraction process is carried out. I have more recently tried truly raw cashews that have been harvested by hand—these are more expensive, taste different, but I have absolutely no problems with them.

The key thing to remember with other nuts is that the salicylate is probably most concentrated in the skin of the nut so, for example, blanched hazelnuts will be lower in salicylate than whole hazelnuts. I do, when I feel like it, use small amounts of nuts. I occasionally make a very weak milk using blanched hazelnuts using 1oz of hazelnuts to 1 pint of water. I also occasionally have roasted peanuts—I simply pop some raw peanuts into the oven on a baking tray for twenty minutes and when they have roasted for twenty minutes or so the red skins fall away when rubbed between your fingers (wait until they have cooled a little).

Oils and Margarine

For me, the food item that has caused me the most problems over the years has been vegetable fat—oils and margarine.

Ideally, cold pressed oils are the safest as virtually all the others will have been treated with antioxidants such as BHA, BHT and TBHQ. Vitamin E is sometimes used as an alternative antioxidant and some people regard these oils as safe. Sadly, that has not been my experience; I do not know if the problem lies in the type of vitamin E used, whether the vitamin has been treated with a preservative or if some chemical is leeching into the oil from the plastic bottles that these type of oils are usually sold in.

I have tried using all the oils that are supposedly low in salicylate and have so far only found unrefined (cold pressed) organic soya oil to be truly low in salicylate. I can tolerate small amounts of unrefined sunflower oil but am not able to use it on a regular basis.

Over the last ten years I have experimented with a range of oils including rice bran, sunflower, rapeseed, and soya oil. What I have found is that the cold pressed ones are too strong in flavour and I honestly think that sunflower is higher in salicylate than the studies have so far indicated. The salicylate level will generally be lower if the oil has been processed but you then risk possible additives in the oil.

I have discovered that many oils, like grains, are high in phenolic acids: "Phenolic compounds have been reported to be present in all vegetable oils".[51] Like with grains, the unrefined versions will potentially be more problematic. Cold pressed oils are usually perceived as being healthier as they have undergone very little processing and I suspect that this lack of refining is what causes problems for some salicylate sensitives. I certainly have had problems with all the low salicylate oils in their cold pressed forms and their more refined versions also. I suspect that the problem has been the amount of phenols in the cold pressed oils and that additives, even if only as a processing aid, in the more refined versions.

Siger et al obtained the highest total phenolic content from pumpkin and hemp oils (2.5 and 2.4 mg/100 g, respectively). Grapeseed oil had the lowest total phenolic compound content (0.51 mg/100 g). The content of those compounds in soy, sunflower, rapeseed, corn, flax, and rice bran oils was at the level above 1 mg/100 g and did not exceed 2mg/100g.[52] In the same way that studies don't agree on the exact amounts of salicylate in food, studies rarely agree on the amount of phenolic acids in oils but the above information provides a reasonable guide.

The oil I currently use is not one you would expect for someone with a salicylate sensitivity but it is working for me—I am using a mild and light olive oil. Yes I know olives are high in salicylate and trust me I cannot tolerate virgin olive oils at all but this one has been processed a little—you can tell this by the taste which is very mild and the aroma (virtually non existent). The oil is sold in glass bottles which is great as I don't have to worry about the plastics leeching. Anyway, we are all different so this may not work for you but if you have tried lots of oils without long term success then this one might be worth a try.

A recent newcomer to our supermarket shelves is Rice Bran Oil which, initially, appears to be a very welcome alternative to the more usual suspects. There have also been quite a number of positive health benefits linked with rice bran oil so it can seem like an even more attractive product to reach for. Beware. Most of the rice bran oil that is readily available is described as being "cold filtered—this does not mean it has been cold pressed. In fact "cold filtered" simply means that in the stage of manufacturing that is filtration they used a cold method. Most rice bran oil is extracted using various types of chemical solvents so may not be quite as healthy a product as you originally thought. The other clue to it not being the same as cold pressed is that it is usually sold in plastic bottles. When rice bran oil first became readily available in the UK I used it very happily until it was rebranded—unfortunately the method of manufacture was also changed and the oil made me quite ill.

I have not found a margarine that is okay; even those with supposedly low salicylate oils often contain natural colours such as annatto and beta-carotene which cause me problems.

Other Food Chemicals

Some salicylate sensitives also react to amines in food and it is certainly worth looking at the list of foods that are high in amines (see Chapter 5) if problems continue or re-emerge once you have been on a low salicylate diet for some time. When I first tried a low amine diet I experienced further improvements but have found, that over time, I am now able to tolerate these.

There is one type of amine that continues to cause me a problem and that is the sort produced by cooking—basically anything that is too browned or gets slightly burned. Avoiding these helps enormously.

Because of the dietary limitations of a low salicylate diet it is possible to eat too much meat and this can lead to build up of certain amines. I have experienced this and the reaction that develops for me is joint pain and stiffness. A couple of weeks on a vegetarian diet usually resolves the problem for me.

The other natural food chemical that can cause problems is Monosodium Glutamate (MSG). MSG occurs naturally in some foods and is also manufactured for use as a flavour enhancer. Problems are most likely to be caused by the latter. Also, if joint problems persist or reappear then it would be worth eliminating and testing the only other food still in your diet that is high in solanine which is potato. For more information on sources of MSG and solanine see Chapter 5.

Packaging

There will be times when you are convinced that something you are eating is bothering you but when you check on the foods you are eating, you simply cannot find anything that is "wrong". Think back and see if you can identify any changes in the packaging of your usual foods.

Methods and types of packaging are continuously changing. Many of these have coatings designed to help keep food "fresh" longer. One of the must common chemicals applied to packaging appears to be methyl salicylate.

Ready Meals

Meals purchased in restaurants, take outs, or as ready meals from supermarkets are always potentially risky as you will not be able to easily calculate the salicylate levels.

The ingredients list can be checked on supermarket meals. In restaurants and take-outs you need to apply some common sense and not order anything highly seasoned and always check with the chef if you are in doubt about anything. Some studies have tried to measure salicylate levels in foods such as curries and pizzas but the results are always very diverse and in the final analysis tell us very little of use. How meals are produced will vary depending on who is cooking and the amount of spices and herbs will never be the same on two dishes from one restaurant let alone dishes with the same name from a number of restaurants.

Soft Drinks

Most soft drinks are not safe because of the added colours and flavourings. Some people can tolerate lemonades that are free from artificial additives—you'll need to try the different brands on the market until you can find one that is safe for you and has an acceptable taste. Be careful if you try cola drinks as the salicylate in these comes from the added flavourings and could be too concentrated for your body to deal with.

Spices

Well, the figures may vary a little but everyone seems to agree that spices are high in salicylate.

It has often been commented on that whilst spices are high in salicylate if you only use a very small amount you should be just fine. In theory that should be the case but spices (and herbs) can contain very concentrated amounts of salicylate so if you experiment do please be very careful.

I have had the occasional Indian meal—sometimes I've survived the experience with minimal effects, other times I have had a full blown reaction that has taken a few days to get rid of so please be careful.

I use small amounts of fresh garlic in cooking and I do sometimes use chilli powder. I had been quite confused as to how I was getting away with eating chilli powder but it could be that the variety I use is lower in salicylate. Interestingly, the Scotter study[53] found very little salicylate in chilli powder.

Sugars and Sweeteners

Sugar can cause problems especially if it is raw cane sugar with minimal refining. Sadly, many people have also reported problems with white granulated sugar (the problem could be with one of the agents used in the refining process).

Although golden syrup has a relatively low amount of salicylate, eating too much over a number of days can lead to problems. I have tried lots of different sugars over the years and now only use an unrefined organic caster sugar. I react badly to maple syrup but am totally okay with agave syrup.

Honey is usually classed as being high in salicylate (the Scotter study[54] had it as low) but I think this does vary enormously from brand to brand. I'm not the world's greatest fan of honey so I've done little experimenting with honey except in respect of manuka honey which I was keen to be able to use because its beneficial health promoting properties. I use an active manuka honey, UMF 15+, whenever I have a sore throat, upset stomach or a problem with my gums or teeth, and sometimes just because I'd like some. As long as I only use the honey occasionally, I don't have any problems with it.

Artificial sweeteners are generally not salicylate based but these are usually highly complex chemicals and, in my opinion, are best avoided. I never used them before and would not consider using them now. Be very cautious about using artificial sweeteners as a substitute for sugar as these are artificial chemicals and your body will have to detoxify and eliminate them.

Sweets (Candies)

Beware of sweets as these can inadvertently be laden with salicylate mimics and also with high salicylate ingredients. Any type that includes a mint flavouring or contains liquorice will also not be safe.[55,56]

Tea and Coffee

There seems to be a general consensus that decaffeinated tea and coffee are reasonably safe for salicylate sensitives. My experience is that the situation is a little less straightforward than that.

The Swain study[57] provides results on various types of tea including basic black teas, Lapsang souchong, Early Grey and Orange Pekoe. All contained more than 1.9mg/100ml except decaffeinated tea which contained only 0.37mg. Methylene dichloride is a solvent that is commonly used in the decaffeination of coffees and teas. Both caffeine and salicylate are readily soluble in it: "Consequently decaffeinated tea contains markedly reduced salicylate compared with tea and decaffeinated coffee is completely devoid of salicylate".[58]

When tea and coffee have been tested salicylate has always been found. Quite often, decaffeinated versions have not been tested so we have very little hard information to go on. Whilst some chemicals may remove salicylate as well as caffeine, the methods used for decaffeination keep changing—not only are different types of solvents used but water/steam methods are also used. I have no way of knowing, except from experience, which coffees and teas are truly low in salicylate.

It is virtually impossible to buy loose decaffeinated tea and the type that comes in bags I do not consider to be safe for anyone with a salicylate sensitivity simply because there are too many potential salicylate mimics in the paper that teabags are made from. I used to be a total tea addict—there was literally always a cup at my side. Rather strangely, when I first came to an understanding about salicylate sensitivity I just gave tea up without any concerns and switched to drinking mainly water. What I've found, as the years have gone by, is that I do sometimes miss having a warm drink so I have experimented and now have the occasional cup of weak tea— no milk.

I use an organically grown loose-leaf tea. I place a little less than a quarter of a teaspoon in a teapot, add enough boiling water to cover the leaves, count to thirty, pour the water down the sink, add sufficient boiling water to the tea leaves for a cup of tea and within a few seconds pour it into a mug. Don't worry I haven't developed some weird tea ritual, the method I describe is a way of decaffeinating tea at home. I find it works and I've never given myself a salicylate reaction from tea when made this way but I only ever have the occasional cup of tea.

The only herbal tea that comes out consistently quite low in salicylate is chamomile. If you choose to drink chamomile tea do please keep a check on how your salicylate levels are doing. It is probably best to restrict the number of cups of tea you have a day and to keep the infusion quite weak.

I avoided coffee at first simply because I never liked it that much but the need for warm drinks had me retrying coffee. I started out with commercial instant brands then changed to ground coffees that could be made in a cafetiere. I have switched brands over the years—not because of taste but because the manufacturers seem to have changed things and where I was once okay with a brand I started noticing that I was experiencing reactions. I now try avoid instant brands.

Some cereal drinks may be okay but do carefully check the ingredients. As most grains are salicylate free you need to be sure that the other ingredients are safe. Watch out for added flavourings and preservatives.

Vegetables

There are some discrepancies between the Swain[59] study and others on the amount of salicylate in certain vegetables. For example, the research by Wood et al found zero amounts of salicylate in aubergine, broccoli and courgette, and very low amounts in cauliflower, cucumber, green pepper, yellow pepper, and lettuce.[60] Scotter et al found higher amounts in frozen peas, yet frozen sweetcorn and frozen broccoli were very low.[61] They also found that fresh tomatoes and carrots had higher salicylate levels than when cooked suggesting that salicylate is lost during the cooking process. Unfortunately we don't know if they used same batch of vegetables for both raw and cooked tests, we also don't know if the peel was removed. It is also the case that the same results did not take place for all vegetables—there was apparently no difference in the salicylate content of fresh and cooked red peppers (both were very low).

Baxter et al tested the levels of salicylic acid in soups made from organic and non-organic vegetables. They found that salicylic acid was present in all of the organic and most of the non-organic vegetable soups. The organic soups had a significantly higher content of salicylic acid.[62] I used to grow my own vegetables but I have found that I am far more likely to experience a reaction to organic vegetables than to those grown commercially.

That was ten years ago and I am now going to totally disagree with the above statement. I now find that I do much better with organic vegetables than non-organic ones. Have I changed? Have the type of pesticides used changed? Have storage, transportation, cleaning and packaging of non-organic vegetables changed? I honestly don't know but I suspect it might be a bit of all three.

My own experiments with different vegetables over the years have consistently shown me that if I eat small amounts of organic vegetables, thought to be high in salicylate, I am generally okay. If I eat the same amount of the vegetable and it is not organic I virtually always have a reaction. I can only suppose that this is in some way linked with residues of pesticide or anti-bacterial washes. One of my experiments that sticks in my mind was that of cauliflower. One year I grew my own and ate quite a number of them during the growing season with absolutely no problems at all. Supermarket bought cauliflower gave me immediate problems and unfortunately even their organic ones caused me problems. Now, I am either an expert at growing low salicylate cauliflowers or the supermarkets are washing the vegetables with something more than water and residues of these chemicals are being left on the vegetables. The only cauliflower that did not bother me, that I did not grow, came from a farmers market.

The amount of salicylate found in tomatoes varies from low to very high. In the early stages of understanding your salicylate sensitivity, it is best to avoid tomatoes completely. I didn't eat a tomato for years but missing them in sauces prompted me to experiment and I now do have tomatoes in my diet but only in small amounts. I generally avoid raw tomatoes unless I have grown them myself and removed the skin. It has been a couple of years since I last grew any but I really did enjoy them but please understand that I only ate a very small amount at any one meal.

Currently I make sauces for pasta and rice dishes that include tomatoes but I only use a single organic tomato in a dish for four people and never add any herbs. Can a single tomato make a difference to the taste of a sauce? Yes, especially if your palette has got used to the total blandness of a diet very low in salicylate. Please note that I only use one organic tomato and I remove the peel. Tip—to peel a tomato place it in a glass jug, cover with boiling water for a couple of minutes, remove with a fork, pierce the skin with a knife and simply peel the skin away.

Don't be tempted to try commercially made sauces as these rely heavily on concentrated amounts of tomato and, usually, large amounts of herbs and/or spices.

It is interesting that Wood et al study[63] found no salicylate in broccoli and the Scotter study[64] found frozen broccoli to be very low. My own experience would not agree with these findings as a full portion of "normal" broccoli gives me a reaction. I do, however, find that small portions of purple sprouting broccoli to be just fine so variety really does seem to make a difference.

My best advice is, when your diet is level, and you know how to clearly spot when your salicylate levels are going too high then experiment with introducing a vegetable you particularly miss. I did this with tomatoes, as described above, and fresh peas—when these are in season I resist the urge to eat them raw but I allow myself a small amount of them when cooked.

Please note that I never eat a number of high salicylate vegetables in a single day. If you decide to experiment make sure you space experiments apart, peel whenever possible, and keep your portion sizes small. If you give yourself a reaction don't worry—at least now you know what it is happening.

Water

By far the safest drink is water. I drink lots of water but even this has not been without its problems for me. Long before the original salicylate handbook I was using water filters for drinking water at home as our water supply, at that time, was highly chlorinated. The filter jug system seemed to work without any problems for me until the company introduced a new set of filters.

It took me quite a few months before I worked out that the problems I was experiencing were linked with the water I was drinking. I stopped using the filters and used only bottled water for a few weeks and everything settled down for me. At that point I opted to buy a water distiller which I have now been using for over two years with great success. I don't know what was being used in the water filter or whether it was something leaching into the water from the plastic container but the filtered water really was a problem for me and this was definitely an example of how difficult it is at times to work out just what is going on. So, if you find yourself getting confused about why you are reacting oddly immediately ask yourself what you have been doing differently since before the symptoms started.

Yeast

Brewer's yeast in the form of tablets, powders or flakes should be avoided because of potentially high amounts of salicylate.[65]

Bekatorou et al note that salicylates, either naturally occurring or added as flavouring agents, may be present in yeast and yeast extracts. The flavouring agents include benzyl salicylate, methyl salicylate, ethyl salicylate, isoamyl salicylate, isobutyl salicylate, and phenethyl salicylates.

Baker's yeast is most usually the strain called saccharomyces cerevisiae. It has traditionally been produced using molasses from sugar industry by products. In theory, therefore, fresh baker's yeast for bread making should be of no concern to anyone with a salicylate sensitivity. Unfortunately, the manufacturing process includes the use of emulsifiers and cutting oils. It is also possible that the processing aids contain salicylate. If you use yeast in baking at home try the various options available to you to see which you are most comfortable with. I bake my own bread using a dried active yeast.

In respect of shop bought bread, you will have no way of knowing if the yeast used contains any salicylate. It is perhaps best to assume that the bread is okay but to remember the above information in case you find yourself experiencing reactions you are unable to explain in any other way.

Food Additives

Some food additives can also be a problem not necessarily because they contain any salicylate but because some of them mimic salicylate in their effect or are similar in chemical structure.

Adverse reactions to tartrazine are common in people who also react badly to salicylate,[66] probably because both are similar in structure and are detoxified in the same way. Similar problems have been found with the antioxidants BHA and BHT.[67] Elverland noted that azo dyes and food preservatives induced similar symptoms to those caused by aspirin intolerance.[68]

Below you will find information on the various categories of additives that can cause problems. By far the easiest course of action is to avoid as many additives as possible especially during the testing phase.

Generally the only way of testing if one is okay with a food additive is to exclude foods that contain the additive(s) and then reintroduce the food and monitor for reactions. Doctors can also test for allergies using skin prick tests. Colour dyes can be tested directly at home if you are able to buy the dye. A study by Stevens et al, in respect of ADHD in children, recommends that small bottles of food dye are purchased and, on a weekend when the parent is at home the child should be asked "to print/or write his name, read aloud from an age-appropriate book, and solve some maths problems. Then, the parent should put a few drops of each color into water or pure fruit juice and ask the child to drink it." After 30 minutes ask the child to do the handwriting etc... again and repeat again 15 minutes later noting any changes that may take place.[69] I'm a little uneasy about testing anything in a concentrated form at home and would advocate checking with your doctor first or testing by removing foods with the colour and then later reintroducing them.

Antioxidants

BHA, BHT and TBHQ are synthetic compounds and do not occur in nature. They were originally developed for use in petroleum and rubber products. When their antioxidant properties were realised they began to be used in foods. BHA is more common than BHT because it offers greater stability at higher temperatures. TBHQ is the new kid on the block but is finding its way into an increasing number of products. Fisherman and Cohen identified cross reactivity between aspirin intolerance and ingestion of BHA and BHT.[70]

You will find that BHA and/or BHT find their way into most refined vegetable oils. Unless an oil is cold pressed it has probably, at some stage, been treated with an antioxidant which is unlikely to appear on the label. You can also be exposed to BHA and BHT via food packaging materials, lubricants and sealing gaskets for food containers.[71] They have also been found in mineral oil products, ointments, cosmetics, chewing gums and medicines. I have also seen mention of BHA and/or BHT in products as diverse as gelatin and pencil tops.

Stokes and Scudder found that the chronic ingestion of 0.5% BHA or BHT by pregnant mice and their offspring resulted in a variety of behavioural changes. Compared to controls, BHA-treated offspring showed increased exploration, decreased sleeping, decreased self-grooming, slower learning, and a decreased orientation reflex. BHT-treated offspring showed decreased sleeping, increased social and isolation-induced aggression, and a severe deficit in learning.[72]

Feingold found that BHT may be incorporated into annatto and beta-carotene colourings used often in products such as cheese and margarine.[73] Please note these are often listed as "natural" colourings and on the surface do seem as if they will be safe but these can often be a source of hidden problems. It is also the case that that BHT and BHA may have been used to preserve vitamins in products such as cereals. Feingold noted that vitamins A, D, and E frequently contain BHT.[74]

In respect of TBHQ, Winter writes: "Death has occurred from the ingestion of as little as 5 grams. Ingestion of a single gram (a thirtieth of an ounce) has caused nausea, vomiting, ringing in the ears, delirium, a sense of suffocation, and collapse. Industrial workers exposed to the vapours, without obvious systemic effects, suffered clouding of the eye lens.[75]

Other antioxidants that may also cause problems are:

E310 Propyl gallate
E311 Octyl gallate
E312 Dodecyl gallate

Benzoic Acid

Benzoic acid occurs naturally in many berries, fruits, herbs and spices (such as cinnamon and cloves), vegetables and tea. The existence of benzoic acid in its natural form has been known since at least the sixteenth century. Today it is commercially manufactured by the chemical reaction of toluene, a hydrocarbon obtained from petroleum, with oxygen in the presence of cobalt and manganese salts as catalysts.

The commercial form is used in the food manufacturing process as a preservative and also has widespread non-food uses. The use of derivatives such as benzoyl peroxide for bleaching flour is an example of how this can become a hidden sensitivity as bleaching agents rarely have to be declared on products they have been used in. The intake levels from natural sources are low in comparison with potential intake levels from food additives.

Reactions to this group of additives have been observed in people with an aspirin or salicylate sensitivity and should be avoided. Benzoic acid has also been found to react with the preservative sodium bisulphite (E222) so sulphites may also be a problem (see *Sulphites* below for a complete list). If you suspect benzoates are a problem, the additives you need to avoid are:

E210 Benzoic Acid
E211 Sodium benzoate
E212 Potassium Benzoate
E213 Calcium Benzoate
E214 Ethyl 4-hydroxybenzoate

E215 Ethyl 4-hydroxybenzoate, sodium salt
E216 Propyl 4-hydroxybenzoate
E217 Propyl 4-hydroxybenzoate, sodium salt
E218 Methyl 4-hydroxybenzoate
E219 Methyl 4-hydroxybenzoate sodium salt

Colours

Cross-reactions have been noted between salicylate, sodium benzoate and tartrazine.[76] Doeglas found that 19 out of 23 aspirin sensitive patients also reacted to one or more of the following: tartrazine, sodium benzoate, 4-hydroxybenzoic acid, sodium and phenyl salicylate and various analgesics.[77]

Tartrazine and benzoates were found to cause headache, migraine, over activity, problems with concentration, learning difficulties, depression, and joint pain.[78]

A Spanish study found that many people sensitive to acetyl-salicylic acid also react to tartrazine. The amount of tartrazine leading to a reaction ranged from minimal amounts up to 750 mg and symptoms appeared anywhere between a few minutes and 14 hours.[79]

Tartrazine, E102, finds its way into a whole host of products and not just food—check all medicines, supplements, toothpastes, mouth washes etc...

A number of other colours, natural and man made, are also potentially a problem and are best avoided. It is hard to know for definite which colours are definitely a problem as the way in which they are produced varies. A list of the most common colours is given below, I tend to avoid them all as I rarely buy foods that have been coloured.

E100 Curcumin
E101 (i) Riboflavin (ii) Riboflavin-5'-phosphate
E102 Tartrazine

E104 Quinoline Yellow

E110 Sunset Yellow FCF, Orange Yellow S

E120 Cochineal, Carminic acid, Carmines

E122 Azorubine, Carmoisine

E123 Amaranth

E124 Ponceau 4R, Cochineal Red A

E127 Erythrosine

E128 Red 2G

E129 Allura Red AC

E131 Patent Blue V

E132 Indigotine, Indigo carmine

E133 Brilliant Blue FCF

E140 Chlorophylis and Chlorophyllins: (i) Chlorophylls (ii) Chlorophyllins

E141 Copper complexes of chlorophylls and chlorophyllins: (i) Copper complexes of chlorophylls (ii) Copper complexes of chlorophyllins

E142 Greens S

E150a Plain caramel

E150b Caustic sulphite caramel

E150c Ammonia caramel

E150d Sulphite ammonia caramel

E151 Brilliant Black BN, Black PN

E153 Vegetable carbon

E154 Brown FK

E155 Brown HT

E160a Carotenes: (i) Mixed carotenes (ii) Beta-carotene

E160b Annatto, bixin, norbixin

E160c Paprika extract, capsanthin, capsorubin

E160d Lycopene

E160e Beta-apo-8'-carotenal (C 30)

E160f Ethyl ester of beta-apo-8'-carotenic acid (C 30)

E162 Beetroot Red

E160a Carotenes: (i) Mixed carotenes (ii) Beta-carotene

E160b Annatto, bixin, norbixin
E160c Paprika extract, capsanthin, capsorubin
E160d Lycopene
E160e Beta-apo-8'-carotenal (C 30)
E160f Ethyl ester of beta-apo-8'-carotenic acid (C 30)
E162 Beetroot Red
E163 Anthocyanines
E180 Latolrubine BK

Natural Colours

It is easy to assume that natural colours will be safe but, unfortunately, the source of these colours and how they are produced can make them unsafe for salicylate sensitives. I have reacted to both annatto and beta-carotene when use used in margarines and cheeses and now avoid products that contain them.

The colour "annatto" is produced from the seeds of the annatto tree (Bixa orellana). It is the thin highly coloured resinous coating that provides the raw material for making the colour annatto. Annatto is leached from the seeds using an extractant which has been made from one or more food-grade materials including various solvents, oils and fats, alkali aqueous and alcoholic solvents.[80]

A quick internet search will find a range of web sites indicating that annatto contains salicylic acid but none of them provide a reference to confirm this and I certainly have not been able to find out if the amount of salicylate would be classed as low or high. Given that annatto is a plant it is not surprising that it contains some salicylate. We don't know if the reactions experienced by salicylate sensitives to annatto are due to natural salicylate or to some form of contamination by a salicylate mimic during processing.

Mikkelsen et al tested for adverse reactions to annatto. Fifty-six individuals suffering from chronic urticaria and/or angioedema were orally challenge tested with annatto extract—the amount used was a dose equivalent to the amount used in 25g of butter. Twenty-six per cent reacted to annatto within four hours. Quite a number of the study participants also reacted adversely to artificial food colours.[81]

Beta-Carotene has been steadily replacing artificial yellow and orange colours and the natural colour annatto in many products. Whilst beta-carotene may be a natural substance extracted from plants, the process of extraction can lead to contamination with undesirable chemicals. I had a quick look at details from manufacturers of beta-carotene as an additive and most of them stated that the extraction method used was solvent based.

Flavourings

When flavours are added to food rarely is information provided as to what the flavouring actually is. It is by far the safest course of action to avoid any food product that has added flavours. A few examples of flavourings that are not safe for the salicylate sensitive follow:

- Benzaldehyde (artificial oil of almond), often used to flavour maraschino cherries.
- Benzyl salicylate, raspberry flavour.
- Ethyl salicylate, used to produce a mild wintergreen flavour.
- Isoamyl salicylate, a bittersweet strawberry flavour used in root beer and fruit and berry flavoured products.
- Methyl salicylate, the wintergreen flavour often found in chewing gums, sweets, and medicines.

- Phenylethyl salicylate, a sweet peach flavour used to create apricot, peach and pineapple flavourings.
- Salicylaldehyde, provides a nutty flavour used in spice flavourings and products.

Methyl salicylate in large doses can also cause problems for those without a salicylate sensitivity. For example, Howrie reported on the case of a 21-month-old boy who ate sweets containing methyl salicylate as a flavouring. The child developed vomiting, lethargy and breathing problems.[82]

One of the most common flavourings used in chocolate is vanillin and sadly this one is also a problem. This artificial vanilla flavouring is manufactured from clove oil (eugenol), from a breakdown product of lignin from a conifer, or using petrochemical raw materials. As cocoa is salicylate free, chocolate is a safe product but only if it contains natural vanilla (try organic brands and you should be safe) or, preferably, is vanilla free.

Other additives

The additives listed below could also cause problems. It is by no means the case that all of these will affect everyone with a salicylate sensitivity but it is worth being aware of them especially when trying to find out the cause of an unexpected reaction.

E330 Citric acid
E331 Sodium citrates (i) Monosodium citrate (ii) Disodium citrate (iii) Trisodium citrate
E332 Potassium citrates (i) Monopotassium citrate (ii) Tripotassium citrate
E333 Calcium citrates (i) Monocalcium citrate (ii) Dicalcium citrate (iii) Tricalcium citrate

E334 Tartaric acid (L(+)-)

E335 Sodium tartrates (i) Monosodium tartrate (ii) Disodium tartrate

E336 Potassium tartrates (i) Monopotassium tartrate (ii) Dipotassium tartrate

E337 Sodium potassium tartrate

E355 Adipic acid

E356 Sodium adipate

E357 Potassium adipate

E380 Triammonium citrate

E440 Pectins (i) pectin (ii) amidated pectin

E471 Mono- and diglycerides of fatty acids

E472a Acetic acid esters of mono- and diglycerides of fatty acids

E472b Lactic acid esters of mono- and diglycerides of fatty acids

E472c Citric acid esters of mono- and diglycerides of fatty acids

E472d Tartaric acid esters of mono- and diglycerides of fatty acids

E472e Mono- and diacetyl tartaric acid esters of mono- and diglycerides of fatty acids

E472f Mixed acetic and tartaric acid esters of mono- and diglycerides of fatty acids

These may not be tolerated if extremely sensitive:

E460 Cellulose (i) Microcrystalline cellulose (ii) Powdered cellulose

E461 Methyl cellulose

E462 Ethyl cellulose

E463 Hydroxypropyl cellulose

E464 Hydroxypropyl methyl cellulose

E465 Ethyl methyl cellulose
E466 Carboxy methyl cellulose, Sodium carboxy methyl cellulose
E468 Crosslinked sodium carboxymethyl cellulose
E469 Enzymically hydrolysed carboxy methyl cellulose

Sulphites

Sulphites are not necessarily a problem but if there is a more general problem with dealing with food chemicals these are best avoided.

E220 Sulphur dioxide
E221 Sodium sulphite
E222 Sodium hydrogen sulphite
E223 Sodium metabisulphite
E224 Potassium metabisulphite
E226 Calcium sulphite
E227 Calcium hydrogen sulphite
E228 Potassium hydrogen sulphite

E150(b) Caustic Sulphite Caramel
E150 Sulphite Ammonia Caramel

References

[1] Annon. Lancet, 1903, 162, 1187.

[2] Duckwall, EW. Canning and Preserving of Food Products with Bacteriological Technique. Pittsburgh printing company, 1905.

[3] Feingold BF. Dietary management of nystagmus. J Neural Transm 1979;45:2:107-15.

[4] Shelley WB. Birch Pollen and Aspirin Psoriasis: A Study in Salicylate Hypersensitivity. JAMA 196428;189:985-8.

[5] Swain A , Dutten SP, Truswell AS. Salicylates in Food. J Am Dietetic Assoc 1985;85(8).

[6] Wood A, Baxter G, Thies F, Kyle J, Duthie G. A systematic review of salicylates in foods: estimated daily intake of a Scottish population. Mol Nutr Food Res. 2011 May;55 Suppl 1:S7-S14.

[7] Scotter MJ, Roberts DPT., Wilson LA, Howard FAC, Davis J, Mansell N. Free salicylic acid and acetyl salicylic acid content of foods using gas chromatography–mass spectrometry. Food Chemistry, Vol 105, 1, 2007, 273-279 .

[8] Swain A , Dutten SP, Truswell AS. Salicylates in Food. J Am Dietetic Assoc 1985;85(8).

[9] Wood A, Baxter G, Thies F, Kyle J, Duthie G. A systematic review of salicylates in foods: estimated daily intake of a Scottish population. Mol Nutr Food Res. 2011 May;55 Suppl 1:S7-S14.

[10] Swain A , Dutten SP, Truswell AS. Salicylates in Food. J Am Dietetic Assoc 1985;85(8).

[11] Wood A, Baxter G, Thies F, Kyle J, Duthie G. A systematic review of salicylates in foods: estimated daily intake of a Scottish population. Mol Nutr Food Res. 2011 May;55 Suppl 1:S7-S14.

[12] Saltmarsh M, Crozier A, Ratcliffe B. Fruit and Vegetables. In: Goldberg G (ed). Plants: Diet and Health (British Nutrition Foundation). Wiley-Blackwell, 2003.

[13] Alonso Garcia A., Cancho Grande B., Simal Gandara J. (2004) Development of a rapid method based on solid-phase extraction and liquid chromatography with ultraviolet absorbance detection for the determination of polyphenols in alcohol-free beers. Journal of Chromatography A 1054:175-180.

[14] Scotter MJ, Roberts DPT., Wilson LA, Howard FAC, Davis J, Mansell N. Free salicylic acid and acetyl salicylic acid content of foods using gas chromatography–mass spectrometry. Food Chemistry, Vol 105, 1, 2007, 273-279 .

[15] Swain A , Dutten SP, Truswell AS. Salicylates in Food. J Am Dietetic Assoc 1985;85(8).

[16] Scotter MJ, Roberts DPT., Wilson LA, Howard FAC, Davis J, Mansell N. Free salicylic acid and acetyl salicylic acid content of foods using gas chromatography–mass spectrometry. Food Chemistry, Vol 105, 1, 2007, 273-279 .

[17] Paterson J, Baxter G, Lawrence J, Duthie G.Is there a role for dietary salicylates in health? Proc Nutr Soc. 2006 Feb;65(1):93-6.

[18] Breakey J. What's Become Of The Feingold Diet? http://www.abc.net.au/rn/science/ockham/stories/s412378.htm.

[19] Breakey J, Hill M, Reilly C, Connell H. Report of a trial of the low additive, low salicylate diet in the treatment of behaviour and learning problems in children. Aust J Nutr Diet 1991;48:89-94.

[20] Janssen PL, Katan MB, Hollman PC, Venema DP. Determination of Acetylsalicylic Acid and Salicylic Acid in Foods, Using HPLC with Fluorescence Detection. J. Agric. Food Chem., 1996, 44 (7), 1762–1767.

[21] Swain A , Dutten SP, Truswell AS. Salicylates in Food. J Am Dietetic Assoc 1985;85(8).

[22] Wood A, Baxter G, Thies F, Kyle J, Duthie G. A systematic review of salicylates in foods: estimated daily intake of a Scottish population. Mol Nutr Food Res. 2011 May;55 Suppl 1:S7-S14.

[23] Scotter MJ, Roberts DPT., Wilson LA, Howard FAC, Davis J, Mansell N. Free salicylic acid and acetyl salicylic acid content of foods using gas chromatography–mass spectrometry. Food Chemistry, Vol 105, 1, 2007, 273-279 .

[24] Wood A, Baxter G, Thies F, Kyle J, Duthie G. A systematic review of salicylates in foods: estimated daily intake of a Scottish population. Mol Nutr Food Res. 2011 May;55 Suppl 1:S7-S14.

[25] Scotter MJ, Roberts DPT., Wilson LA, Howard FAC, Davis J, Mansell N. Free salicylic acid and acetyl salicylic acid content of foods using gas chromatography–mass spectrometry. Food Chemistry, Vol 105, 1, 2007, 273-279 .

[26] Wood A, Baxter G, Thies F, Kyle J, Duthie G. A systematic review of salicylates in foods: estimated daily intake of a Scottish population. Mol Nutr Food Res. 2011 May;55 Suppl 1:S7-S14.

[27] Swain A , Dutten SP, Truswell AS. Salicylates in Food. J Am Dietetic Assoc 1985;85(8).

[28] Wood A, Baxter G, Thies F, Kyle J, Duthie G. A systematic review of salicylates in foods: estimated daily intake of a Scottish population. Mol Nutr Food Res. 2011 May;55 Suppl 1:S7-S14.

[29] Scotter MJ, Roberts DPT., Wilson LA, Howard FAC, Davis J, Mansell N. Free salicylic acid and acetyl salicylic acid content of foods using gas chromatography–mass spectrometry. Food Chemistry, Vol 105, 1, 2007, 273-279 .

[30] Ibid.

[31] Wood A, Baxter G, Thies F, Kyle J, Duthie G. A systematic review of salicylates in foods: estimated daily intake of a Scottish population. Mol Nutr Food Res. 2011 May;55 Suppl 1:S7-S14.

[32] Kim KH, Tsao R, Yang R, Cui SW. Phenolic acid profiles and antioxidant activities of wheat bran extracts and the effect of hydrolysis conditions. Food Chemistry, Vol 95, 3, April 2006, 466-473.

[33] Dykes L, Rooney LW. Phenolic compounds in cereal grains and their health benefits. doi:10.1094/CFW-52-3-00105. 2007.

[34] Mattila P., Kumpulainen J. (2002) Determination of free and total phenolic acids in plant-derived foods by HPLC with diode-array detection. Journal of Agricultural and Food Chemistry 50:3660-3667.

[35] Zielinski H., Kozlowska H., Lewczuk B. (2001) Bioactive compounds in the cereal grains before and after hydrothermal processing. Innovative Food Science and Emerging Technologies 2:159-169.

[36] Kato H., Ohta T., Tsugita T., Hosaka Y. (1983) Effect of parboiling on texture and flavor components of cooked rice. Journal of Agricultural and Food Chemistry 31:818-823.

[37] Sosulski F., Krygier K., Hogge L. (1982) Free, esterified, and insoluble-bound phenolic acids. 3. Composition of phenolic acids in cereal and potato flours. Journal of Agricultural and Food Chemistry 30:337-340.

[38] Ibid.

[39] Ibid.

[40] Kim KH, Tsao R, Yang R, Cui SW. Phenolic acid profiles and antioxidant activities of wheat bran extracts and the effect of hydrolysis conditions. Food Chemistry, Vol 95, 3, April 2006, 466-473.

[41] Kato H., Ohta T., Tsugita T., Hosaka Y. (1983) Effect of parboiling on texture and flavor components of cooked rice. Journal of Agricultural and Food Chemistry 31:818-823.

[42] Dykes L, Rooney LW. Phenolic compounds in cereal grains and their health benefits. doi:10.1094/CFW-52-3-00105. 2007.

[43] Duke JA. Handbook of phytochemical constituents of GRAS herbs and other economic plants. Boca Raton, FL. 1992, CRC Press.

[44] Tay SY, Tham E, Yeo CT, Yi FC, Chen JY, Cheong N, Chua KY, Lee BW. Anaphylaxis following the ingestion of flour contaminated by house

dust mites--a report of two cases from Singapore. Asian Pac J Allergy Immunol. 2008 Jun-Sep;26(2-3):165-70.

[45] Sánchez-Borges M, Suárez-Chacon R, Capriles-Hulett A, Caballero-Fonseca F, Iraola V, Fernández-Caldas E. Pancake Syndrome (Oral Mite Anaphylaxis). WAO Journal: May 2009, Vol 2, 5, 91-96.

[46] McGee H. McGee on Food & Cooking. Hodder & Stoughton, 2004.

[47] Süss A, Rytter M, Sticherling M, Simon JC. Anaphylactic reaction to soy drink in three patients with birch pollen allergy. J Dtsch Dermatol Ges. 2005 Nov;3(11):895-7.

[48] De Swert LF, Gadisseur R, Sjolander S, Raes M, Leus J, Van HE. Secondary soy allergy in children with birch pollen allergy may cause both chronic and acute symptoms. Pediatr Allergy Immunol 2011 Oct 21.

[49] Ping L., Xu-Qing W., Huai-Zhou W., Yong-Ning W. (1993) High Performance Liquid Chromatographic Determination of Phenolic Acids in Fruits and Vegetables. Biomedical and Environmental Sciences 6:389-398.

[50] Ross, IA. Medicinal Plants of the World, Volume 2. Humana Press, 2001.

[51] Siger A, Nogala-Kalucka M, Lampart-Szczapa E. The content and antioxidant activity of phenolic compounds in cold pressed plant oils. Journal of Food Lipids, 15: 137–149.

[52] Ibid.

[53] Scotter MJ, Roberts DPT., Wilson LA, Howard FAC, Davis J, Mansell N. Free salicylic acid and acetyl salicylic acid content of foods using gas chromatography–mass spectrometry. Food Chemistry, Vol 105, 1, 2007, 273-279 .

[54] Ibid.

[55] Beckstrom-Sternberg, Stephen M., and James A. Duke. "The Phytochemical Database." http://ars-genome.cornell.edu/cgi-bin/WebAce/webace?db=phytochemdb. (Data version July 1994).

[56] Swain A , Dutten SP, Truswell AS. Salicylates in Food. J Am Dietetic Assoc 1985;85(8).

[57] Swain A , Dutten SP, Truswell AS. Salicylates in Food. J Am Dietetic Assoc 1985;85(8).

[58] Ibid.

[59] Ibid.

[60] Wood A, Baxter G, Thies F, Kyle J, Duthie G. A systematic review of salicylates in foods: estimated daily intake of a Scottish population. Mol Nutr Food Res. 2011 May;55 Suppl 1:S7-S14.

[61] Scotter MJ, Roberts DPT., Wilson LA, Howard FAC, Davis J, Mansell N. Free salicylic acid and acetyl salicylic acid content of foods using gas chromatography–mass spectrometry. Food Chemistry, Vol 105, 1, 2007, 273-279 .

[62] Baxter G J, Graham A B, Lawrence J R, Wiles D, Paterson J R. Salicylic acid in soups prepared from organically and non-organically grown vegetables. Eur J Nutr 2001;40(6):289-92.

[63] Wood A, Baxter G, Thies F, Kyle J, Duthie G. A systematic review of salicylates in foods: estimated daily intake of a Scottish population. Mol Nutr Food Res. 2011 May;55 Suppl 1:S7-S14.

[64] Scotter MJ, Roberts DPT., Wilson LA, Howard FAC, Davis J, Mansell N. Free salicylic acid and acetyl salicylic acid content of foods using gas chromatography–mass spectrometry. Food Chemistry, Vol 105, 1, 2007, 273-279 .

[65] Bekatorou, A. Psarianos, C. Koutinas, A.A. Production of food grade yeasts Food Technology and Biotechnology 44 (3) , 407-415 2006.

[66] Settipane GA, Pudupakkam RK. Aspirin intolerance III: sub-types, familial occurence and cross reactivity with tartrazine. J Allergy Clin Immunol 1975;56:215-21.

[67] Fisherman EW, Cohen GN. Aspirin and other crossreacting small chemicals in known aspirin intolerant patients. Ann Allergy 1973;31:476-84.

[68] Elverland HH. Sensitivity to acetylsalicylic acid. Tidsskr Nor Laegeforen 1996,28;116(6):754-6.

[69] Stevens LJ, Kuczek T, Burgess JR, Hurt E, Arnold LE. Dietary sensitivities and ADHD symptoms: thirty-five years of research. Clin Pediatr (Phila). 2011 Apr;50(4):279-93.

[70] Fisherman EW, Cohen GN. Aspirin and other crossreacting small chemicals in known aspirin intolerant patients. Ann Allergy 1973;31:476-84.

[71] Weber RW. Adverse reactions to the antioxidants butylated hydroxyanisole (BHA) and butylated hydroxytoluene (BHT). In: Metcalfe DD, Sampson HA, Simon RA. (eds) Food Allergy: Adverse reactions to foods and food additives, 2nd ed. Blackwell Science 1997:387-95.

[72] Stokes JD, Scudder CL. The effect of butylated hydroxyanisole and butylated hydroxytoluene on behavioral development of mice. Dev Psychobiol 1974;7(4):343-50.

[73] Feingold B, Feingold H. The Feingold Cookbook for Hyperactive Children and others with problems associated with food additives and salicylates. Random House, 1979.

[74] Ibid.

[75] Winter, RA. Food Additives: A consumer's dictionary. Three Rivers Press, 1999, fifth edition.

[76] Settipane GA. Aspirin and allergic diseases: a review. Am J Med 1983;74(6A):102-9.

[77] Doeglas HM. Reactions to aspirin and food additives in patients with chronic urticaria, including the physical urticarias. Br J Dermatol 1975;93(2):135-44.

[78] Novembre E, Dini L, Bernardini R, Resti M, Vierucci A . Unusual reactions to food additives. Pediatr Med Chir 1992;14(1):39-42.

[79] Alvarez Cuesta E, Alcover Sanchez R, Sainz Martin T, Anaya Turrientes M, Garcia Rodriguez D. Pharmaceutical prepartions which contain tartrazine. Allergol Immunopathol 1981;9(1):45-54.

[80] Lucas CD, Hallagan JB, Taylor SL.The role of natural color additives in food allergy. Adv Food Nutr Res. 2001;43:195-216.

[81] Mikkelsen H, Larsen JC, Tarding F. Hypersensitivity reactions to food colours with special reference to the natural colour annatto extract (butter colour). Arch Toxicol Suppl. 1978;(1):141-3.

[82] Howrie DL, Moriarty R, Breit R Candy flavoring as a source of salicylate poisoning. Pediatrics 1985;75(5):869-71.

3 Non-Food Sources

Sadly, salicylates can be found in a whole range of everyday products and, depending on your sensitivity, you will have to watch out for them. Not everyone who reacts to salicylate in food also reacts to these non-food sources but familiarising yourself with the potential risks of these products may save you from being thrown by an unexplained reaction.

The results of research carried out in 1989 by Williams et al support the theory that some industrial chemicals induce intolerance because of their aspirin-like properties.[1] The main ways in which you are likely to come into contact with these sources of salicylate, and salicylate mimics, is through contact with the skin or by inhalation.

Absorbed and airborne salicylate cause problems in different ways than ingested salicylate. Absorption through the skin will usually, but not always, produce a rash and that is sufficient warning that there is a problem with the product so continued use can be avoided. Inhaled salicylate, in my experience, can cause a reaction far more speedily than that caused by food—reactions usually take place within minutes (with some symptoms appearing over the next 12 hours). The severity and length of these reactions seems to depend on a range of factors including how much other salicylate you currently have in your system, how well you are and how you respond to the reaction.

If you are feeling sceptical and believe that if a product is on the market then it must be safe just remember that the most commonly available form of salicylate is aspirin and that aspirin intoxication can and does lead to death. Also, recently the UK government withdrew a commonly used disinfectant from the National Health Service due to the number of adverse reactions being experienced by staff—mainly skin and breathing problems.[2] I doubt that we were ever intended to inhale, absorb and ingest the cocktail of chemicals currently found in our air, food and medicines and it really is no wonder that people experience problems with dealing with these.

There is little specific research on salicylate in non-food sources and its role in health has not really been explored. I have tried to pull together the main categories of products/substances that can cause problems as a guide. I have also included, in Appendix 2, a list of chemical names but the information below and in the lists will only help you in a limited way because most of these non-food products do not carry a list, partial or full, of ingredients. You will have to learn to trust your instincts, and your nose, as to the safety of many products. One of the easiest ways forward is to go as perfume and chemical free as possible—it is a challenge at first but it does get easier.

Salicylates through the Skin

Many ointments especially anti-inflammatory ones contain some form of salicylate. The purpose of these is to ensure that the active ingredient (salicylate) is delivered directly to the problem area. The extent to which these are absorbed into the blood and redistributed throughout the body is still not wholly known but the cases below demonstrate how easily a salicylate overdose can take place in people who are not diagnosed as having a salicylate sensitivity.

A 1996 study by Morra et al concluded that a considerable amount of salicylic acid may be absorbed through the skin after using products containing methyl salicylate and that this may increase with regular use.[3] We know, that after application, large quantities can be measured in the skin and tissue and that salicylate, once absorbed into the blood, passes freely around the body.[4] Perry et al have estimated that 12-20% of the salicylate in skin preparations is absorbed and given that some ointments contain up to 40g of salicylate per 100g a significant amount can be absorbed.[5] They stress the need to avoid these in cases of salicylate sensitivity.

Salicylate absorption through the skin can lead to serious problems. Pertoldi et al describe the case of a 70-year-old man with psoriasis which was being treated with a cream containing salicylic acid. After five days of using the cream the man was admitted to ICU with encephalopathy (various neurologic symptoms including changes in consciousness, behaviour and personality changes) and severe acid-base disturbances including respiratory alkalosis and metabolic acidosis. It would appear that, as this man's skin was damaged with the psoriasis, the salicylate was absorbed at a greater rate than it would ordinarily have been. The authors suggest that anyone (salicylate sensitive or not) being prescribed topical salicylate treatments should routinely have their blood salicylate levels monitored which is, currently, far from being a common practice.[6]

Pec et al describe a case where a man treated his psoriasis with a 40% salicylic ointment. Nineteen hours after the application his blood salicylate level had reached excessive levels and the man needed hospitalisation for fourteen days.[7] Raschkeet al describe a case of severe hypoglycaemia which a man experienced after using a topical salicylate to treat psoriasis.[8] Use of ointments containing salicylate for the treatment of psoriasis have also led to the development of tinnitus.[9]

Hausen and Schulz found that the dye used in stockings and hose can affect individuals sensitive to those dyes.[10]

Germann et al describe the case of a 7 year old boy who experienced life threatening salicylate poisoning as a result of the ointment being used to treat his icthyosis vulgaris (very dry scaly skin condition) over a period of four weeks. The child had experienced wheezing, vomiting, tinnitus, vertigo and fell into a state of unconsciousness. It was six months after the incident before the neurological problems, including problems with the eyes, that he was experiencing finally cleared up.[11]

Topical salicylic acid is used widely in wart removal applications. The reactions that some people experience can be much more widespread than inflammation of the skin. Laraschi et al present the case of a nine-year-old boy who started with abdominal pain, nausea, constipation, increasing weakness and general illness after two days of using patches with 15% salicylic acid for a plantar wart. Various tests were carried out with no success. The wart treatment continued for a month and the symptoms improved only when the patches were removed—within a few days, the symptoms had abated. The patches were retried and within two days the symptoms reappeared. A full recovery was made once the use of the patches was stopped, and all the symptoms had disappeared within two weeks.[12]

A forty-five year old man sought advice after two weeks of increasing pain and swelling in his left hand. The symptoms arose after using an ointment that was 12% salicylic acid. He applied the cream more often than the instructions advised. When the area around the wart became painful and swollen, his doctor prescribed antibiotics. After ten days of taking these without benefit he attended the accident and emergency department. Tests identified that whilst he had chronic inflammation there was no infection. Treatment included a split skin graft and the man had to spend two weeks in hospital. It was determined that the severe chemical reaction was as a result of "overzealous application" of the salicylic acid cream.[13]

It is quite likely that, if you are salicylate sensitive, an application of an ointment containing some form of salicylate will result in skin irritation. If this takes place you would be advised to avoid the product. If there is no skin irritation then closely monitor your health to see if there is delayed reaction—remember that salicylate is cumulative in the body and symptoms appearing on one day are more likely to be related to something you did a few days ago.

Ensure that none of the high and very high foods, especially herbs and spices, are present in any ointment you use and avoid any that contain an ingredient that has the terms "salicylate", "salicylic" or "Sali" within it. Also, be very careful about checking for additives such as colours and antioxidants. Back in the early days of understanding salicylate sensitivity I used an antifungal cream on a tiny patch of athletes foot—after a few days of use my toes had swollen so much I could not get shoes on or walk without great discomfort. A large part of my foot had become red and inflamed and it wasn't until I stopped using the cream that the problem began to go away—the cream contained BHA.

Inhaled Salicylate

The human nose can distinguish more than 10,000 odours.[14] For something to have an odour it must contain some combination of chemicals and it is when this combination includes a form of salicylate that problems can arise.

My own experience is that inhaled reactions produce some symptoms immediately or within minutes. If I find myself coughing, retching and unable to catch my breath there's no doubt that I have been "got" and that other symptoms will follow. I've found as the years have gone by that this almost violent reaction has reduced in its intensity. I sometimes race out of a highly scented place desperate for air and cough a little but I haven't been reduced to a total state for some time. That is not to say that I don't get reactions from airborne salicylate because I still do but these are no longer as severe. I have also got much better at avoiding having them.

Unfortunately sometimes the first indication I have that something is not right is when I realise I have visual or auditory distortion. I can also become confused, disorientated and other worldly. I can only imagine that a young child experiencing something similar would be quite distressed and unable to let you know what was happening. The good news is that the worst usually passes within 30-40 minutes. One thing I have learnt over the years is not to get into a car until the worst has passed—when your vision becomes distorted it can seem as if every car in the opposite lane is coming straight at you. So once again parents please note that rushing to get your child home may not always be the right thing to do—I would suggest a walk in fresh air and something to eat in case there has also been a blood sugar dip.

Unfortunately it is impossible to predict how toxic any particular place is going to be. My motto regarding airborne salicylate is quite simply "if in doubt get out". I always carry a handkerchief that I can place over my mouth and breath through for those times when I walk into a haze of perfume in a shop or other public place. I also now always use a personal air purifier in public places. I've used one of these for a few years now and have at times doubted whether it was doing anything useful. Those doubts have evaporated when, on occasion, I haven't realised that the battery has died and have started to feel quite ill or unable to breath easily in shops. I also carry a facemask primarily for use in public toilet facilities—the use of highly perfumed detergents and air fresheners seems to be increasing and some of these make me very sick. I have also been known to wear the mask in shops that have displays of scented candles.

Airborne salicylate can come from natural sources such as plants, herbs and their oils; and from man made chemicals.

Shelley notes that the only trees which produce methyl salicylate in levels to be readily detected by the nose are sweet birch, black birch and to a lesser extent yellow birch.[15] Wintergreen (teaberry) is the only shrub with this property. It is thought that the pollen of wintergreen, Spiraca, and the willows present a low risk because the size is small, the trees are few in number and pollination is carried out by bees. Salicylate has been identified in birch pollen and can cause serious problems for someone sensitive to it.[16] Eriksson found a correlation between birch pollen allergy and a sensitivity to many fruits and nuts.[17] It is possible that the common link between these is salicylate, as many fruits and nuts are high in salicylate.

"Spices and flavoring agents contain volatile essential oils and hydrocarbons which stimulate glandular secretion and may have a weak action on the nervous system".[18] I certainly find some essential oils more problematic than others. I have no problems with the smell of oils like lavender, orange, and lemon but experience an instant reaction to oils like clove, wintergreen and thyme.

The increasing interest in aromatherapy has presented a further natural inhalation hazard as these are very concentrated sources of salicylate and, these days, are found in shops, offices and homes.

Dahleen found bronchial absorption of aspirin after inhalation of lysine-aspirin in both asthmatic and non asthmatic subjects.[19]

Crinon in an article on the health effects of airborne solvent exposure tells us that chemicals known as solvents are part of a broad class of chemicals called volatile organic compounds.[20] These compounds are frequently used in a variety of settings and off-gas readily into the atmosphere. As a result of their overuse, they can be found in detectable levels in virtually all samples of both indoor and outdoor air. Once in the body they can lead to a variety of neurological, immunological, endocrinological, genitourinary, and hematopoietic problems. Some individuals also have metabolic defects that diminish the liver's clearing capacity for these compounds. Unfortunately, solvents reach a point at which they do not release a detectable odour but that does not stop them from causing problems if inhaled.

Perfumes and solvents can give you reactions and it is very difficult to know if they contain salicylate or not. The only way of knowing is to trust your instincts as well as your nose, which at first can lead to many unwanted reactions. If it all sounds difficult then you're reading the situation correctly. The positive side, and it is a massive one, is the better health that follows. Salicylate causes so many problems within the nervous system that all aspects of your life are affected by it— reducing the level substantially can, for someone with a salicylate sensitivity, lead to many positive changes.

See the sections below for further details in particular read the section on fragrances.

Potential Problems

Below you will find details of some potential problem areas. Inevitably there will be others but hopefully by familiarising yourself with the ones below you will know what type of thing to look out for especially when trying to identify the cause of a reaction.

Air Fresheners

The number of air fresheners in use seems to have increased alarmingly—everywhere you go there seems to be one and they get into your clothes and hair as well as your lungs.

If you have any of these at home, whether they are plug in, spray, sit on the surface, in the form of a candle, or whatever form they come in, get rid of them. Your body needs fresh air not chemicals—open some windows.

If you have a problem with unwanted odours explore the option of air purifiers—the number of these that are available increases each year and you can find ones that are very, very quiet. There are also some chemical free odour removers on the market.

Benzoates and Parabens

Benzoates, in their various forms, creep into many non-food products and can cause problems for anyone with a salicylate sensitivity.

Esters of para-hydroxybenzoic acid, more commonly known as parabens, are used widely in medications and cosmetics. In fact, benzoates can be found in a variety of non-food products including medicines, perfumes, cosmetics, toothpaste, lice treatments, resin preparations, in the production of plasticisers, in dyestuffs, synthetic fibres, as a chemical intermediate, as a corrosion inhibitor in paints, a curing agent in tobacco, as a mordant in calico printing and in insecticides. Some exposure may also result from inhalation of auto exhaust, tobacco smoke and other combustion sources.

Cars

Remove any air fresheners and don't try replace these with anything else except more regular car cleaning and when cleaning stick to using water and vinegar or water and sodium bicarbonate on the inside. The outside if washed at a commercial car wash is probably okay as long as it is not you that has driven the car through—airborne chemical odours will permeate inside. Formulations for windscreen wash bottles can be hazardous and anti-freeze sprays may also cause problems—we now resort to scraping, and using only water, to remove ice.

Be wary of allowing family members to give lifts to anyone who uses a large number of scented products either on themselves or on their clothing—these permeate into the upholstery and can cause problems for weeks after.

New cars have been treated with many chemicals and could be a source of problems for some.

Taxis (cabs) are a hazard that I had not thought of until one day, out of necessity, I had to use one. I had the reaction from hell as a result of that five minute ride and that was despite having explained to the driver I was having a problem and had him open all the windows and placed a mask over my face. I'm afraid I simply reacted too late and the hanging tree air freshener "got" me.

Fragrances

Fragrances that can cause problems can be both natural (essential oils and spices) and synthetic. The natural ones are relatively easy to avoid as they are usually clearly labelled but synthetic ones that are a problem are less easy to identify. Sadly, today, synthetic chemicals are the ones most widely used.

In many products such as air fresheners or perfumes you will not know if the scent is natural or not but if it smells like a suspect salicylate (for example, almond, clove, mint, orange, strawberry) then avoid it.

Essential oils are a hazard and not just some of the most obvious ones: For example, amber has isoamyl salicylate as one of its constituents, carnation and ylang ylang contain methyl salicylate. It is safest to avoid them all. Salicylates are also commonly used as fixatives—substances added to perfumes to make them last longer.

A few examples of salicylate in fragrances follow:

Amyl salicylate (Pentyl Ortho Hydroxy Benzoate) has a sweet, herbaceous, slightly floral odour. It is used as a solvent for synthetic musks and as a fixative in floral compositions such as jasmine, lilac, and lily.

Benzaldehyde (artificial oil of almond) is one of the base compounds in many perfumes.

Benzyl benzoate itself has very little odour but is often used to improve the odour characteristics of other more costly ingredients.

Benzyl salicylate(2-Hydroxybenzoic acid, phenylmethyl ester; Benzyl ortho hydroxy benzoate) is used as a floral balsamic odour and also as a blender and fixative.

Veratraldehyde has a vanilla odour and is mixed with vanillin to make scents.

It is exceedingly difficult to avoid fragrances but, at least within the home, you can eliminate them—no perfume, no after shaves, no scented toiletries such as antiperspirants, shampoos and soaps, and no scented household products such as cleaning fluids, air fresheners, washing powders, and candles. You will greatly reduce the toxic load that your body has to contend with by removing these from your home.

Gardening

Gardening is a definite hazard. Always wear gloves to prevent too much skin contact. I had a particularly unpleasant experience after cutting back a gooseberry bush; having climbed underneath it, contact had been made with my head and arms and the end result was the nastiest doze of hives I have ever experienced. Since then I have maintained a respectful distance from any plant that needs a lot of work doing to it but find that all other activities are quite safe as long as I wear gloves and a long sleeved shirt.

It is impossible to provide a complete list of plants that contain salicylate but some of the more common ones are:

Acacia, American Pennyroyal, Aspen, Birch, Camelia, Cananga, Clove, Gaultheria, Geraniums, Goosefoots, Hyacinth, Lilies, Magnolia, Marigolds, Meadowsweet, Milkwort, Mints, Poplar, Rose hips, Teaberry, Tulips, Viola, Violets, Willow, Wintergreen.

Be cautious when using chemicals of any sort in the garden. Pesticides, fertilisers, insecticides, patio cleaners and similar type products could all be a potential problem so check and if in doubt don't use them.

Herbal Medicines

Given the high levels of salicylate that have been found in the herbs that have been analysed, it is by far the safest option to avoid herbal remedies. If you decide to try some please be aware that, because of the paucity of information on salicylate levels in herbs, an inexperienced herbalist could unwittingly prescribe herbs that are not safe for a someone with a salicylate sensitivity.

A further area of concern is in the possible adulteration of herbal remedies. Phua et al note that herbal medicines do not usually provide immediate relief of symptoms "as most of them are generally concerned with homeostasis" and advice that if a remedy comes with claims of providing immediate relief of symptoms it should be treated as potentially suspect as it may contain non-herbal preparations:

> A survey in Taiwan found that 23.7% of 2,609 herbal samples had been adulterated with pharmaceuticals.

> A study of 243 products in California found that 7% contained undeclared pharmaceuticals.

They note that the most common pharmaceuticals used in this way are non-steroidal anti-inflammatory drugs (NSAIDs) and anti histamines.[21] DasGupta found that some herbal preparations have been adulterated with medicines including acetyl salicylate (aspirin).[22]

The risk of salicylate from herbal preparations is not the only one of concern, if the herbs are not organic there may very well be some form of salicylate in the pesticides that have been used.

If you feel you have to use a herb whether it is for cooking or as a supplement/treatment then treat it as suspect and start with very small amounts. Here are some of the herbs I know contain salicylate:

> Acacia,[23] Alfalfa, Aloe Vera,[24] Apocynaceae,[25] Birch, Black haw,[26] Chamomile, Cramp bark,[27] German Sarsaparilla, Gingko Biloba,[28] Jasmine,[29] Magnolia, Meadowsweet, Poplar,[30] Purple Loosestrife, Silver Birch,[31] Sweet Birch, White and Red Flower oils,[32] Willow, Woodlock oils.

Others that I have seen mentioned as containing salicylate include:

Astragalus, Borage Oil, Echinacea, Evening Primrose, Ginseng, Goldenseal, Horsetail Extract, Kava Kava, Milk Thistle, Nettle, Passion Flower, Rosemary, St Johns Wort, Valerian.

A number of herbs, such as Echinacea, Aloe Vera, Valerian, Evening Primrose, Borage and Astragalas, have become quite popular but, for the salicylate sensitive individual, it is safest to avoid any preparation containing herbs. Herbal remedies are often ingested in a very concentrated form and as the greater majority of herbs that were tested in the Australian study[33] were found to be very high in salicylate I believe it is safest to avoid as many herbs as possible.

As many people now use herbs as an alternative to drug treatment this is a major blow. As we do not know if all herbs contain salicylate, or what the amount within them is, any degree of experimentation could be potentially harmful. If you really feel you must use herbal remedies then consider using tinctures in which the herb has been greatly distilled. Remember that salicylate builds up in the system so monitor your health very carefully. Dried herbs or herb teas could make you very ill—under no circumstances test these when on your own.

Herbs in ointment are also risky and any prolonged use will increase the overall amount of salicylate in your body, occasional use, for most people, will probably be okay but NOT if there is an immediate reaction such as a rash or itching.

Occasionally suffering from a bad back I found myself completely thrown by not being able to use standard back rub ointments as they are all laden with camphor and methyl salicylate—the smell of which is enough to bring on unwanted symptoms. I resorted to using alternating cold and hot compresses and the occasional application of a comfrey ointment.

Household Products

You need to suspect any household product that contains a fragrance. They do not all contain salicylate but it is impossible to know which do and which do not. By far the safest way forward is to remove all scented products from the house.

It is not difficult to remove products such as air fresheners and scented candles but some products are essential to every day living like washing up liquids, washing powders and general cleaning fluids. The only advice I can give is find the simplest and purest brand you can. Some companies do now provide safer more environmentally friendly products and if you can find one that is fragrance free then use that one.

I have not eliminated all scented products from our house but I have changed every single one of them. It took a little time of eliminating and trying new ones until I found ones that were less harmful than others. An example of this is that washing clothes without some fabric conditioner proved unacceptable—the static, regardless of what I did, was extreme. For a number of years, I compromised and used very, very small amounts of a "natural" conditioner that did contain some scent but was not as heavily laden as most commercial brands.

As a rule of thumb I avoid anything that has been coloured. I have found that the scents used in clear or white liquids seem to be less salicylate laden than their coloured counterparts but this is by no means a fool proof test. These days I simply apply a sniff test and know immediately if a product is safe for me or not. In the early days it was a question of removing and then trying a new product and monitoring any reactions.

Unless you are certain that fragrances are a concern I would suggest you begin the elimination process slowly. Start with the room that you sleep in and clear it of any scented products—potpourri, air fresheners, essential oils etc... Clean the room with unscented products only and remove clothes that have been worn (scents build up in the fabrics) or washed in scented products. If you begin to notice a difference then tackle the rest of the house.

It is amazing how far one can get by using a solution of sodium bicarbonate or vinegar in water when cleaning. I have also found that bleach (unscented) causes me no problems and is very useful for bathroom use.

Be aware that it is not only scented products that are a source of concern. Some others such as insecticides and glues can also cause difficulties. If someone in your house is a hobbyist who uses glues then ask them to try solvent free varieties.

Is this beginning to sound impossible to deal with? If it is I know how you feel. I remember being totally overwhelmed and also of making many mistakes. The key word is "simplicity". Begin to reduce the number of chemicals in your house and all the family will benefit—each of these chemicals that we inhale or absorb through our skin has to be dealt with by the body. Products that need to be "reviewed" include:

Air fresheners, Anti-mildew spray, Candles, Detergents, Fabric Conditioners, Floor Cleaners, Furniture Polishes, Glues, Insecticides, Lubricating oils, Paint, Soap Pads, Toilet Cleaners, Washing Powders, Washing up Liquids, Window Cleaners.

Other items may also cause problems such as certain inks used in printing, fibre tips pens, rubber or plastic products that have been sealed for a long time such as mouse mats and cool bags (these can sometimes out gas so leave them in a garage or shed), dried flowers.

New clothing, bedding, and curtains should always be washed before being worn/used to remove chemicals residues from treatments and scents that have impregnated the fabrics whilst on display in the shops.

New furniture can also be a hazard—be prepared for a problem and never bring into the house a whole range of new products at one time. All of these products will have been treated in some way and some, not all, of these chemicals can cause problems. New carpeting and flooring and the adhesives used with these can also cause problems

When it comes to decorating choose wallpaper that can be stuck with solvent free adhesives, and paints that are as low in odour as possible (there are also some solvent free paints now available). Only have decorating carried out when the weather is warm enough for extremely good ventilation and try get the work completed as fast as possible. If your sensitivity is very extreme you may need to leave the house whilst this work is being carried out and use an air filter for the following few weeks.

I have changed the products that I use many times over the years and it is heartening to see the emergence of many more fragrance free products. Some of the products that I currently use:

Washing Powder: For hand washing I use soap flakes. In the washing machine I now use Lakeland's Laundry Balls. I no longer use a fabric conditioner.

Washing up Liquid: Earth Friendly's Dishmate (Fragrance free).

General Cleaning: Most microfiber cloths work just great without anything else.

Cream Cleaner: Ecover Cream Cleaner.

Window Cleaner: Earth Friendly's Window Cleaner (vinegar or lavender).

Medicines

All forms of aspirin and NSAID's (non-steroidal anti-inflammartory drugs) need to be avoided. Do not make the assumption that it is only painkillers or anti-inflammatory drugs that contain salicylate. Sadly it creeps into a whole range of drugs that are used to treat different conditions including:

Acne treatments
Anti-acids
Antiseptics/disinfectants
Colitis drugs (Mesalamine contains 5-aminosalicylic acid)
Corn and Wart removers
Cough Medicines
Foot powders
Mouth Washes and gargles
Mouth Ulcer preparations
Ointments for treatment of psoriasis, eczema, and dermatitis.
Ointments for joint and back pain
Teething gels

I have decided not to supply a list of drugs that contain salicylate in whatever form as no such list could be wholly comprehensive and would not be applicable to all countries. Always, always check with your doctor and/or pharmacist about any drug treatment whether prescribed or over the counter and don't forget about the non active ingredients such as binders, colours and antioxidants—non active ingredients such as BHA, BHT, flavourings, benzoates, tartrazine and other colours can also be found in medicines.[34]

In respect of pain relief most salicylate sensitives are okay with acetaminophen (Paraecetmol/Tylenol) but please be aware that there have been cases reported of people reacting to both aspirin and acetaminophen.[35] The reason for this could be that aspirin is a cyclooxygenase inhibitor; Schwarz and Ham Pong note that it "has been reported that acetaminophen may in high doses crossreact with aspirin due to weak cyclooxygenase inhibition".[36]

My own experience is that prolonged use of acetaminophen (for example, during bouts of flu) leaves me with a sensation of having been "got". It is not a salicylate reaction as such but I feel slightly poisoned and "not right". A couple of days without any rectifies the problem and occasional usage has never caused me a problem. Please remember we are all different—what is safe for me may not be safe for you. Beware of liquid forms as these often contain added colours.

Acetylsalicylic acid and other salicylates are known to cross react with other drugs most notably NSAIDs. You should always check and double check with your doctor and pharmacist before agreeing to take any medication. Kurowski and Brune list a number of drugs that interact in some way with salicylate including acetazolamide, methrotexate, penicillin, secoborbital, and warfarin.[37] Please note that all drugs affect each other in some way and simply because a drug has certain effects when taken in conjunction with aspirin does not mean that it will be unsafe for you if you are salicylate sensitive. Check with your doctor.

Pesticides

Methyl salicylate is one of the most common additions to a wide range of products ranging from chewing gum wrappers to cartons for storing clothes:

> "The pesticidal uses of methyl salicylate include vertebrate repellent on terrestrial and greenhouse food crops and as an insect repellent when incorporated into a coating on the internal and outer surfaces of cartons used to store consumer products like human and pet foods, animal feeds and nonfood items such as clothing and textiles."[38]

I have also seen mentions of methyl salicylate washes for fruit and vegetable during storage which may explain why fruit and vegetables that are supposedly low in salicylate, such as pomegranate, can sometimes appear not to be.[39]

It is impossible to avoid all forms of salicylate but it is useful to have an overview of the type of places that they can crop in so that you can help understand some of the strange reactions you may experience that simply don't make sense.

Products for babies and very young children

Assume that everything may be a problem. Unfortunately, many of the products that state they are natural can also be a problem if they contain too many natural herbal essences in them.

Some of the items that need careful checking include:

Teething gel, cough remedies, shampoo, soap, creams and lotions, wet wipes, and disposable diapers.

Sunscreens

I have not been able to find a sunscreen that is salicylate free.

Ironically, during my experimenting phase I experienced worse reactions to some brands of fragrance free hypoallergenic brands than to certain scented ones. This is because some of the basic ingredients of sunscreens are salicylate based. Homosalate (hommenthyl salicylate), octyl and benzyl salicylate are frequently used for their properties as UV-B blockers and because they help moisturise the skin. Other ingredients are not immediately recognisable as salicylate but many have similar chemical structure and need to be avoided.

The list of salicylates in sunscreens is long. They are used as UV absorbers and filters, solvents, fixatives and invariably make an appearance in the fragrances. Some of the more common ones are listed below:

Acetyl salicylic acid
Aluminium acetyl salicylate
Ammonium salicylate
Benzyl salicylate
Calcium acetyl salicylate
Choline salicylate
Ethyl salicylate
Ethylhexyl salicylate
Glycol salicylate
Isopropyl salicylate
Lithium salicylate

Methyl salicylate
Para amino salicylic acid
Phenyl salicylate
Procaine salicylate
Sal ethyl carbonate
Salicylamide
Salicylic acid
Sodium salicylate
Stroncylate
Strontium salicylate

I have not been able to find a safe alternative. What I find works for me is to limit to my direct exposure to the sun as much as possible. If I have to be out in the hottest part of summer days (we don't have too many of these in England so the problem is not too great) I wear a wide brimmed straw hat, cotton dresses, skirts or trousers and a long sleeved cotton shirt.

I never suspected that my sensitivity to the sun was in any way linked with my salicylate sensitivity but I have discovered that it is known that magnesium salicylate can increase sensitivity to sunlight. Whether other forms of salicylate do the same is can is not recorded but my own experience would indicate that they probably do—suddenly one summer I seemed to have fewer problems than ever before. Exposure with no sunscreens or additional cover up clothes took far longer (hours) before I began to feel ill; prior to my low salicylate existence, it would take a few minutes at most. I've noticed, over the years, that when I am unwell due to an excess of salicylate in my system I have a much lower tolerance to the sun than when my salicylate level is low.

Toiletries and Cosmetics

The more scented the product, the greater the risk. It is best to avoid using perfume and scented products. All of the following potentially contain some form of salicylate.

Contact lens cleansers, cosmetics, creams and ointments, denture fixatives, deodorants, hair dyes, hair sprays and gels, lip balms, make up, mouth wash and gargles, toothpaste, teething gels, shaving foams, skin and hair conditioners, soap, and shampoo.

Fragrance and colour free products are increasingly available but do check the labels for other forms of salicylate, buy the smallest size available and test it.

Products that reduce dry skin should be checked very carefully as they often contain beta hydroxy acids (BHAs) which are made up of mainly salicylic acid and its derivatives. Beware medicated shampoos as these often contain salicylate. Hair conditioners are often full of salicylate in particular butyloctyl salicylate, alkyl salicylate, hexyldodecyl salicylate and isodecyl salicylate.

Soap, shower gels and shampoos are often laden with colours and scents and frequently contain Amyl Salicylate, Benzyl Salicylate, Hexenyl-3-Cis Salicylate, and Hexyl Salicylate.

A further group of chemicals you need to watch out for are parabens which creep into many cosmetic type products and can cause problems for the salicylate sensitive. The easiest way to deal with these is to remove all scented and most coloured products.

Our bathroom shelves now have very few products. I have tried various shampoos over the years and it has been heart breaking when a much appreciated brand suddenly stops being produced or the ingredients get altered. A couple of years ago I was forced into trying to find an alternative and after some unpleasant experiments with fragrance free shampoos that were simply too high in glycerine I tried some commercial brands with disastrous results. The hair care market keeps changing with new wonder treatments and products and some of these are lethal. I was ill for days after trying a commercial shampoo and even worse I couldn't remove the smell——it was in my clothes, pillows, upholstery. I landed up having to take a steam cleaner to the furniture, buy new pillows and cut my hair very short as I simply could not remove the smell.

The end-result of the last bout of hair shampoo experiments was to try a totally natural product—rhassoul clay. You place some powdered rhassoul clay into a pot add some water, leave to activate and then rub into your wet hair, leave for a couple of minutes and rinse out. I love it, it keeps my hair clean and shiny.

Soap has, also, at times shown itself to be a challenge. There are some basic fragrance free bars on the market that most supermarkets stock. I currently am using Sonett curd soap (not very easy to find in the UK) but am looking for a new type as I find the glycerine content a little too high.

For years I used only sodium bicarbonate as a substitute for toothpaste but I'm thrilled with a new toothbrush—the Soladey toothbrush which relies on light and your own saliva to do the cleaning.

Deodarants are easy to replace. If you really want to use a commercial type then there are lots of fragrance free ones on the market. An alternative is to use a mineral based one such as Pit Rok's Natural Crystal Stick which is what I am currently using.

In respect of make-up, I wrote in 2002 "I have experimented with make up and have found that some brands are okay but the ingredients in these products change with alarming regularity so you would need to check very carefully if you wish to use it—I gave up". I'm pleased to report that the last few years have seen various mineral based make-ups arrive on the market. I still don't wear them very often but I do now have a range of these mineral based products and have found them to be safe (please note that I have not tested any lipsticks).

In 2002, I noted that one of the most frustrating things for me was a search for a moisturising cream and in the end I gave up and used soya oil instead which worked well enough as it did not leave a greasy residue. I have tried various commercial products since then.

There are some fragrance free creams on the market that are probably okay I just don't like them. I land up being concerned about some of the chemicals in them and then, just as I've got used to them, the company seems to change the ingredients they use. The more natural ones are often combined with something that isn't okay—for example, many cocoa butter creams are combined with almond oil. Newer butters to the market such as shea butter have not worked for me. I now make my own cream using cocoa butter and grapeseed oil.

Others

It would be impossible to provide a comprehensive list of all the products and ways in which salicylate appears but some of the others are mentioned below. Hopefully, these combined with the information above will give you an idea of the multitude of ways in which you come into contact with salicylate and lessen your anxiety when seemingly inexplicable reactions take place.

Benzyl alcohol finds its way into products such as colour photography and contact lens cleaners.

Certain printing inks often on full colour brochures are a problem.

Benzaldehyde which appears in food flavourings and perfumes is also used in the pharmaceutical industry and in the production of plastics. It is also used as a raw material for the production of other products including benzyl alcohol, benzyl amine, dibenzyl amine, hexyl and amyl cinnamic aldehydes and cinnamic aldehyde.

Finger paints and play-doughs used by children are likely to contain colours and possible other chemicals—these substances could be introduced into the mouth by hands and fingers.

Salicylate creeps into illegal drugs, it has been found to be present in some forms of ecstasy tablets.[40] Given that users of these often take multiple pills the salicylate alone could prove fatal for an individual sensitive to it.

Products containing balsam of peru, propolis.

Salicylic acid is in many countries permitted as a preservative in adhesives used for food packaging, in paperboard containers which will be in contact with foods, and for closures for sealing gaskets of food containers.

Fire wood from birch and willow trees.

Salicylate Free Products

The number of these on the market has increased primarily because of interest in a particular form of treatment for fibromyalgia sufferers that involves eliminating use of salicylate in certain forms.

When I have checked the ingredients lists of many of these products there is no way that I, as a salicylate sensitive, would risk them—quite a few of them are high enough in salicylate or salicylate mimics to make me very ill. So, if you want to try these be cautious and remember that most of these have not been produced for people who have a salicylate sensitivity. Things do change and we may soon have some products that are truly salicylate free so do keep checking.

References

[1] Williams WR,Pawlowicz A, Davies BH. Aspirin-like effects of selected food additives and industrial sensitising agents. Clin Exp Allergy 1989;19(5):533-37.

[2] BBC News: Disinfectant withdrawn over safety fears. 22 Jan 2002. http://news.bbc.co.uk

[3] Morra P, Bartle WR, Walker SE, Lee SN, Bowles SK, Reeves RA. Serum concentrations of salicylic acid following topically applied salicylate derivatives. Ann Pharmacother 1996;30(9):935-40.

[4] CSPI booklet 'A Parent's Guide to Diet, ADHD, and Behavior', 1991.

[5] Perry CA , Dwyer J, Gelfand JA, Couris RR, McCloskey WW. Health effects of salicylates in foods and drugs. Nutrition reviews 1996;54(8):225-240.

[6] Pertoldi F, D'Orlando L, Mercante WP. Acute salicylate intoxication after trancutaneous absorption. Minerva Anestesiol 1999;65(7-8):571-3.

[7] Pec J, Strmenova M, Palencarova E, Pullmann R, Funiakova S, Visnovsky P, Buchanec J, Lazarova Z. Salicylate intoxication after use of topical salicylic acid ointment by a patient with psoriasis. Cutis 1992 Oct;50(4):307-9.

[8] Raschke R, Arnold-Capell PA, Richeson R, Curry SC. Refractory hypoglycemia secondary to topical salicylate intoxication. Arch Intern Med 1991;151(3):591-3.

[9] Maune S, Frese KA, Mrowietz U, Reker U. Toxic inner ear damage in topical treatment of psoriasis with salicylates. Laryngorhinootologie 1997;76(6):368-70.

[10] Hausen BM, Schulz KH. Allergy to dye in stockings. Dtsch Med Wochenschr 1984;109(39):1469-75.

[11] Germann R, Schindera I, Kuch M, Seitz U, Altmeyer S, Schindera F. Life threatening salicylate poisoning caused by percutaneous absorption in severe ichthyosis vulgaris. Hautarzt 1996;47(8):624-7.

[12] Loraschi A, Marelli R, Crema F, Lecchini S, Cosentino M. An unusual systemic reaction associated with topical salicylic acid in a paediatric patient. Br J Clin Pharmacol. 2008 Jul;66(1):152-3.

[13] Tavakkolizadeh A, Povlsen B. A serious complication of topical wart treatment on the hand. J R Soc Med. 2004 Apr;97(4):180.

[14] Kochhar KP. Dietary spices in health and diseases: I. Indian J Physiol Pharmacol. 2008 Apr-Jun;52(2):106-22.

[15] Shelley WB. Birch Pollen and Aspirin Psoriasis: A Study in Salicylate Hypersensitivity. JAMA 196428;189:985-8.

[16] Ibid.

[17] Eriksson NE. A relationship between food sensitivity and birch pollen-allergy and between food sensitivity and acetylsalicylic acid intolerance. Allergy 1978;33(4):189-96.

[18] Kochhar KP. Dietary spices in health and diseases: I. Indian J Physiol Pharmacol. 2008 Apr-Jun;52(2):106-22.

[19] Dahlen B, Boreus LO, Anderson P, Andersson R, Zetterstrom O. Plasma acetylsalicylic acid and salicylic acid levels during aspirin provocation in aspirin-sensitive subjects. Allergy 1994;49(1):43-9.

[20] Crinnion W J. Environmental Medicine, Part 2 - Health Effects of and Protection from Ubiquitous Airborne Solvent Exposure. Altern Med Rev 2000;5(2):133-143.

[21] Phua DH, Zosel A, Heard K. Dietray supplements and herbal medicine toxicities—when to anticipate them and how to manage them. Int J Emerg Med (2009) 2:69-76.

[22] DasGupta, A. Effects of Herbal Supplements on Clinical Laboratory Test Results (Patient Safety). Walter de Gruyter & Co, 2011, 99.

[23] Shelley WB. Birch Pollen and Aspirin Psoriasis: A Study in Salicylate Hypersensitivity. JAMA 1964, 28;189:985-8.

[24] Klein AD, Penneys NS. Aloe vera. J Am Acad Dermatol. 1988 Apr;18(4 Pt 1):714-20.

[25] London, A., Veres, K., Szabo, K., Haznagy-Radnai,E., Mathe, I. Analysis of the essential oil of Amsonia illustris. Nat Prod Commun, February 1, 2011; 6(2): 235-6.

[26] Cabrera, C. Fibromyalgia: A Journey Toward Healing: A Journey Towards Healing. McGraw-Hill Contemporary, 2002.

[27] Ibid.

[28] Ross, IA. Medicinal Plants of the World, Volume 2. Humana Press, 2001.

[29] Behl, P.N Skin-Irritant and Sensitizing Plants found in India. Chand, 1979.

[30] Cabrera, C. Fibromyalgia: A Journey Toward Healing: A Journey Towards Healing. McGraw-Hill Contemporary, 2002.

[31] Ibid

[32] DasGupta, A. Effects of Herbal Supplements on Clinical Laboratory Test Results (Patient Safety). Walter de Gruyter & Co, 2011, 107.

[33] Swain A , Dutten SP, Truswell AS. Salicylates in Food. J Am Dietetic Assoc 1985;85(8).

[34] Bhatia MS. Allergy to tartrazine in psychotropic drugs. J Clin Psychiatry 2000;61(7):473-6.

[35] Schwarz N, Ham Pong A. Acetaminophen anaphylaxis with aspirin and sodim salicyalte sensitivity: a case report. Ann Allergy, Asthma, Immunol 1996;77:473-474.

[36] Ibid.

[37] Kurowski M, Brune K. Other unwanted side effects and drug interactions with aspirin and other salicylates. In: Aspirin and Other Salicylates. Ed Vane JR, Botting RM. Chapman and Hall 1992, 576-599.

[38] METHYL SALICYLATE PC Code 076601. Reregistration Eligiblity Document. US Environmental Protection Agency Office of Pesticide Programs. September 27, 2005.

[39] Sayyaria M, Babalare M, Kalantarie S, Serranoc M, Valerod D. Effect of salicylic acid treatment on reducing chilling injury in stored pomegranates. Postharvest Biology and Technology, Vol 53, 3, 2009, 152-154.

[40] Baggott M et al. Chemical Analysis of Ecstasy Pills: Research Letter. JAMA 200;284:17.

4 Causes and Theories

Causes

Why some people develop a sensitivity to salicylate is not known. We do know that it is not an allergy in the conventional meaning of the word, i.e. a sensitivity that can be measured in the blood using standard IgE testing.

In a research paper on adverse reactions to foods, Allen et al point out that since the discovery of IgE in the mid 1960s the focus of interest in adverse reactions swung towards allergy being the main cause. They write that it is becoming increasingly clear that other mechanisms are responsible in the overwhelming majority of cases.[1] What these other mechanisms are is as yet unknown but it is most definitely the case that you can react severely to either foods or food chemicals and have completely negative allergy tests.

They make the observation that, for many people with a food intolerance, the problem is not so much the food as the chemicals, such as salicylate, within the food—the reactions being pharmacological rather than immunological in nature. The end result for many individuals is that the symptoms are very similar, if not the same, as if they had had an allergic reaction. Similar findings were made by Patriarca et al when they investigated aspirin intolerance. They used acetylsalicylic acid, aspiryl-polylysine, lysine acetyl salicylate, and sodium salicylate in their tests and in only a few individuals was there an immunological response.[2]

Lessof also refers to adverse reactions to salicylates in food as pharmacological reactions rather than immunological ones.[3] Sainte-Laudy arrives at a similar conclusion that despite manifesting as an allergic response aspirin intolerance is not an allergy in the sense that it cannot be measured by IgE testing.[4]

The age at which reactions takes place seems to vary although I suspect that this has more to do with the age at which the sensitivity is diagnosed rather than the actual start of the sensitivity. Speer et al did note that women of childbearing age are especially prone to developing aspirin sensitivity, otherwise the age of onset is approximately equal in the two sexes, varying from one year to sixty years.[5]

The theory of it being an inherited condition does not appear to be backed up by current research. For example, in respect of aspirin induced asthma only a very small number of cases were found to have a family history of a similar intolerance.[6]

Salicylate in the Body

Salicylates produce a wide range of toxic effects that are related to your age, the amount of salicylate you have ingested, absorbed or inhaled, and the length of exposure time.

Salicylate stimulates the central nervous system. At first this can seem like a burst of energy but then usually leads to feeling disassociated, vague and confused. It can bring on tinnitus, headaches and upset stomachs. If inhaled, the breathing can be constricted and lead to retching and dizziness.

The metabolic effects lead to excess CO_2 which stimulates breathing (salicylates on their own also stimulate breathing). The end result can be a condition known as respiratory alkalosis. Your kidneys compensate for this apparent alkalosis by excreting bicarbonate accompanied by sodium, potassium and water, in the urine. Dehydration can result, but more importantly, the loss of bicarbonate diminishes the buffering capacity of the body and allows the development of a metabolic acidosis

Salicylate causes your body to burn more glucose and O2 resulting in heat production, glucose consumption, O2 consumption, and CO2 production. The end result of these effects is an increase in body temperature, blood sugar problems which can persist for several days,[7] and a range of biochemical events happen that lead to acidosis. Your lungs try to help by exhaling CO2 but can only do so much and the kidneys become affected. Children are less able to cope with this process than adults are.

The bloodstream carries chemicals around the body and into the brain. In the brain "toxic" chemicals interfere with the chemical and electrical functioning of the brain cells.

Reactions are delayed when the clearance systems become saturated and excess salicylate remains in the system. In respect of poisoning with medicines these delays can be for up to 72 hours before the levels of salicylate are measurable as being "unsafe".[8] So, don't delay if you know you have had an exposure take the remedies available to you immediately and do not wait for the symptoms to actually appear.

If nothing is done to counteract this process then the symptoms will continue until the salicylate is excreted from the body and the amount of time this will take will depend on your individual system and also whether any further salicylate is introduced.

Theories

The cause or causes of salicylate intolerance are not known. The effects on different parts of the body seem to be brought about by different metabolic processes so that information on how salicylate is metabolised in the body provides us with some clues. The key points are outlined below.

We know that about 50-80% of salicylate in the blood is bound by protein while the rest remains in the active, ionised state; protein binding is concentration-dependent. Saturation of binding sites leads to more free salicylate and increased toxicity.[9]

Approximately 80% of small doses of salicylic acid are metabolised in the liver. Conjugation with glycine forms salicyluric acid and with glucuronic acid forms salicyl acyl and phenolic glucuronide. These metabolic pathways have only a limited capacity. Small amounts of salicylic acid are also hydroxylated to gentisic acid.

Salicylates are excreted mainly by the kidney as salicyluric acid (75%), free salicylic acid (10%), salicylic phenol, and acyl glucuronides and gentisic acid. When small doses (less than 250 mg in an adult) are ingested, all pathways proceed by first order kinetics, with an elimination half-life of about 2-3 hours.[10] When higher doses of salicylate are ingested, the half-life becomes longer (15-30 hours) because the biotransformation pathways concerned with the formation of salicyluric acid and salicyl phenolic glucuronide become saturated.

Renal excretion of salicylic acid becomes increasingly important as the metabolic pathways become saturated, because it is extremely sensitive to changes in urinary pH above pH6. The use of urinary alkalinisation exploits this particular aspect of salicylate elimination.

High doses of salicylate cause stimulation followed by depression of the central nervous system. Confusion, dizziness, delirium, psychosis, asterixis, stupor and coma occur usually when metabolic acidosis is the dominant acid-base abnormality. These features are thought to be due to reduced ionisation of salicylic acid and a shift of salicylate from plasma into the brain. Dominant metabolic acidosis is common in young children who are therefore more likely to experience serious intoxication at relatively low plasma salicylate concentrations.[11]

It would appear that ingested salicylate (usually from food and herbs) is processed by the liver and salicylate that is absorbed through the skin is processed by the kidneys. I have also seen it indicated that salicylate, if not converted by the liver, remains in the system in a free state and it is this form that particularly causes problems when it passes into the brain. Free salicylate must be eliminated by the kidneys and this can only take place if the conditions are right.

One of the interesting things that seems to take place when families change their diets to accommodate a salicylate sensitive is that other family members experience improvement in symptoms they had not particularly been aware of before.[12,13] I tentatively suggest that these findings go towards supporting my theory that our bodies are simply not designed to deal with additives and excessive amounts of natural food chemicals.

It is known that the use of aspirin during pregnancy can have an effect on the unborn child.[14] What is not known is the exact nature of these effects. Could it be possible that some children are born with so much salicylate in their systems that they become unable to deal with it? Some children who, without low salicylate and additive free diets, have serious problems seem to grow out of the condition as they get older. Have their bodies simply developed or "recovered" and become more able to eliminate salicylate and salicylate mimics?

Sinusitis may be caused because salicylic acid can accumulate in the synovial fluids and is cleared much more slowly from these than it is from plasma.[15] If the amount of salicylate reaches "irritant" level for the individual then symptoms will appear.

The theory that acetylsalicylic acid inhibits cyclo-oxygenase which catalyses formation of prostoglandins has also been put forward as one of the mechanisms involved in aspirin sensitivity particularly in the way it affects asthma.[16]

High doses of salicylate cause release of adrenaline from the adrenal medulla; this is thought to be partly responsible for the hypoglycaemia that sometimes occurs.[17]

Salicylates block vitamin K, which impacts magnesium levels, which increase adrenaline flow. The increased adrenaline flow then results in a variety of hyper excitability disorders including ADHD.

Miller describes a condition known as "Toxicant-induced loss of tolerance" or TILT which is a two stage disease process.[18]

> Firstly, certain chemical exposures, such as indoor air contaminants, chemical spills, or pesticide applications, cause some people to lose their previous natural tolerance for common chemicals, foods, and drugs.

Secondly, following this, previously tolerated exposures trigger symptoms.

Reactions and responses are individual specific and the condition will invariably be difficult to diagnose but may be the underlying cause of a number of conditions such as chronic fatigue, fibromyalgia, migraines, depression, asthma, multiple chemical sensitivity, and ADHD.

One other explanation that has been suggested is what is known as poor sulphoxidation ability. It would appear that some people have a deficit of a metabolic enzyme called phenol sulfotransferase (PST). PST is used by the body in a number of ways including firstly, in the digestive system to breakdown phenolic compounds in foods (salicylate is a phenolic compound), and secondly, in the brain to remove "used" neurotransmitters. So if an individual is low in PST or perhaps consumes large amounts of high phenolic compounds then its is possible that there is not enough PST left to do the clean-up work in the brain which will mean that the brain will not function effectively. It also seems to be the case that salicylate may reduce PST levels even lower. If this is the case then it could explain why salicylates affect the mind and behaviour.

A study by Alberti et al of metabolic dysfunction in autistic children concluded that the inability to effectively metabolise compounds such as phenolic amines which are toxic for the central nervous system could exacerbate autistic behaviour.[19] Bamforth et al found that certain additives could inhibit certain metabolic actions. For example, tartrazine and vanillin were found to be inhibit dopamine sulphotransferase.[20]

Glutathione-S-transferase (GST) activity in the brain was found to be inhibited by, among other compounds, salicylate.[21] McFadden suggests that impaired sulfation may be a factor in the success of the Feingold diet which reduces the number of phenolic compounds in the diet. Scadding et al found poor sulphoxidation ability in 58 out of 74 patients and suggest that metabolic defects could be part of the cause of adverse reactions to foods.[22]

An increase in urinary methyl histamine has sometimes been noted and has been linked with an increase in the production of leukotriene B4 and/or leukotrienes C4, D4 and E4.[23] Various other theories related to phenols and eicosanoids and how they are used in the body have also been put forward.

To date, the theories go some way to explaining what may be taking place in the body when it receives too much salicylate but we are not really any further along the way to understanding why some individuals have an apparently lower tolerance level for salicylates than others.

"Treatment"

There is no treatment as such for a salicylate sensitivity. Minimising the amount you take in and finding your dietary tolerance level are the main ways of reducing the impact and avoiding problems. Below I outline some ways in which you may be able to help minimise the severity of the sensitivity or the worst effects of the reactions.

Please, please, do get medical advice before attempting any of them. Remember everything interacts with everything else and you don't want to run the risk of trying a home based remedy without knowing that it is safe for you.

For some individuals with aspirin induced asthma and rhinosinusitis desensitisation treatments have met with some success but urticaria induced by aspirin does not respond in the same way.[24] The technique does not appear to have been tried in respect of dietary salicylate problems.

Acid-Alkaline Balance

Salicylate clearance from the body is strongly dependent on pH. For example, if urinary pH increases from 5 to 8, the amount of salicylate eliminated in the urine increases from 3% to more than 80%.[25,26]

Salicylates are excreted mainly by the kidney as salicylic acid, salicyluric acid, salicylic glucuronides and gentisic acid. The proportion excreted of each metabolite, depends upon urinary pH. With urinary alkalinisation, salicylic acid excretion is enhanced.[27]

Drugs and foods that raise urine pH will increase renal clearance and urinary excretion of salicylic acid, thus lowering plasma levels; acidifying drugs or foods will decrease urinary excretion and increase plasma levels.

Apparently, if kidney function is normal, about half of a large dose of salicylate would be excreted within 15-30 hours. As urinary excretion is more rapid if the urine is alkaline, the one "remedy" that I have found most useful, in the early days of my sensitivity, was an alkalising formula that is a mix of sodium and potassium bicarbonate. If there is any form of kidney problem taking this alkalising formula may be dangerous so check with your doctor first. I used to use a product called Alka Clear from the UK company Higher Nature; unfortunately when I last checked I found it contains carrageenan which may be problematic for some salicylate sensitives.

The need to alkalise is further important because many adverse reactions often lead to the body generally becoming more acidic.[28] Eating as many safe fruit and vegetables will assist in maintaining a more alkaline system. These days I use carbonated water with a few of drops of lime juice to help the process along.

Anti Histamines

As a general rule these are unlikely to help but a study by Stevenson et al did find that the asthmatic response of some to acetylsalicylic acid could be due to a release of histamine into the system.[29] I did use anti histamines in the early days with some degree of relief but stopped once I understood my sensitivity more fully. Your doctor will be able to advice on these.

Calcium Gluconate

Tetany, hyper-excitability of nerves and muscles due to decrease in concentration of extracellular ionised calcium, is experienced by some and it has been suggested that it may be corrected with the use of calcium gluconate.[30]

Fluid Increase

After an exposure to too much salicylate you may need to increase your fluid intake as oliguria (secretion of a diminished amount of urine in relation to the fluid intake) sometimes occurs, which is mostly due to dehydration.[31] If this is not treated it can feel like you have developed cystitis.

Glutathione

We know that salicylate is a depletor of glutathione and a lack of glutathione means that the kidneys will find it harder to eliminate salicylate.[32] Will supplementing with glutathione help?

My own experience with this is inconclusive. I tried using L-Cysteine (often regarded as a safer form of glutathione supplementation) but after a few days felt strange and discontinued using it on a regular basis. I don't know whether my "reaction" was simply part of the detoxification process or whether it was a reaction to the L-Cysteine itself. At one point, I did find taking 1-2 capsules, in the immediate 24 hours after a severe reaction, helpful in minimising the severity of the symptoms. I can't remember why I stopped using it—it was possibly because my reactions became less severe and didn't happen as often.

Homeopathy

Homeopathy is a system of medicine that is not accepted by many but it has helped me enormously in reducing the worst effects of many symptoms which is why I mention it here.

A homeopath would take a full history from you and probably prescribe what is known as a "constitutional" remedy which is designed to work on your whole system. There are also remedies that may help with particular symptoms. For example, I have found "Apis mel" (6c or 30c) extremely useful in helping reduce angioedema and brain fogging. A single dose of the homeopathic remedy "Salicylic Acid" (LM 1) after ingesting a large amount of salicylate seems to stop a severe reaction in its tracks. Biochemic Tissue Salts can also be of benefit: in this range I have used "Nat Phos" when dealing with acid reflux, and "Nat Mur" mixed with a little water and applied to rashes is great at relieving itching. I also homeopathic ointments, in particular "Arnica" for bumps and bruises, and "Hypercal" for cuts and sores.

One of the reasons I turned to homeopathic remedies is that they are safe—the active ingredient is present in such small quantities that adverse reactions are pretty much unknown. If you find you are unable to use the remedies because they are usually dispensed in lactose do try a homeopathic pharmacy as liquid remedies in an alcohol base are available (the alcohol can be evaporated by placing the dose in a small amount of hot water and leaving for a few minutes).

Fish Oil

Healy et al present details of three people with salicylate intolerance—their symptoms included severe urticaria and asthma. After supplementing the diet with 10g daily of fish oils rich in omega-3 PUFAs for 6-8 weeks all three experienced complete or virtually complete resolution of symptoms. Symptoms reappeared when the dose was reduced.[33]

I know this study sounds great but it did only apply to three people and was never repeated. Anecdotal evidence seems to suggest that some salicylate sensitives do experience some benefit from supplementing with fish oil. The majority don't and have usually said that the oil makes them feel ill in some way after a few days—the reason has usually been put down to amines or some other food chemical but it is possible that fish oil simply doesn't work and supplies the body with too much of something hence the negative reaction.

Vitamins and Minerals

If you have struggled with a salicylate sensitivity for a long time and not known about it then you may have vitamin deficiencies.

In an article on drugs producing vitamin deficiencies, Montenero notes that usually a drug has a "devitaminizing" action with respect to a single vitamin.[34] Salicylate, however, reduces the levels of vitamins C, K and pantothenate (B5). There is no currently available research to indicate whether a sensitivity to salicylates in food has the same effects.

Vitamin K

Vitamin K is a fat-soluble vitamin that plays an important role in blood clotting and has been linked with calcium use in bone formation. Deficiencies of vitamin K include a wide variety of bleeding disorders, osteoporosis and fractures.

A study by Binkley et al suggested strongly that most American diets contain insufficient vitamin K for adult needs.[35] Joss and LeBlond found that even small doses of methyl salicylate in ointments can affect the efficiency of other drugs; they cite a case in which they suspect that warfarin action was increased by the methyl salicylate affecting vitamin K metabolism.[36]

Long term use of aspirin may increase the need for vitamin K. Salicylates increase the risk of haemorrhage; Treib et al found that salicylates can induce haemorrhage by inhibiting platelet aggregation and, particularly in higher doses, by vitamin K antagonism, leading to severe problems with blood clotting.[37]

The major sign of deficiency is easy bruising. The primary source of vitamin K in the body is that made by the bacteria in the intestines with the remainder coming from food. Major food sources include green leafy vegetables, such as spinach, green cabbage, kale, Swiss chard, turnip greens, broccoli, tomatoes, liver, lean meats, and dairy products.

I would focus on having a healthy system rather than supplementing with vitamin K. If you decide to take extra vitamin K please check with your doctor as, whilst the general advice is that it is safe, there can be side effects. I experienced flushing, sweating, and disorientation within a few days of using a vitamin K2 supplement.

Folic Acid

Deficiencies in folic acid have been found when aspirin has been used, particularly in individuals with rheumatic conditions and those with arthritis.[38,39,40]

Inoue and Walsh describe a case in which aspirin was added to phenytoin treatment for an individual with epilepsy. Within four months there was a folate deficiency.[41]

Vitamin C

Vitamin C deficiency may include bruising, fever, anaemia, emotional changes, swollen and bleeding gums, fatigue, lethargy, jaundice (yellowing of the skin and eyes), increased susceptibility to infections, slow wound healing, and swelling of the lower limbs. Severe deficiency leads to scurvy (rare these days). Use of aspirin would appear to reduce the amount of vitamin C available in the body and can lead to deficiency problems.[42] Ten years ago most people thought that taking extra Vitamin C would help with a reaction but current thinking may indicate the opposite to be true.

The advice on the use of vitamin C with aspirin and other similar medications varies greatly (and keeps changing). The current view appears to be as follows: the body has to breakdown aspirin to remove it and large amounts of vitamin C might decrease the breakdown of aspirin. Decreasing the breakdown of aspirin might increase the effects and side effects of aspirin. So, the advice currently is, do not take large amounts of vitamin C if you take large amounts of aspirin.[43] Does the same problem take place with large amounts of salicylate from food? We don't know but I think we have to assume that there is some similarity and that high doses of vitamin C, in the form of a supplement, combined with a meal high in salicylate is probably best avoided.

In a few years time, new research may indicate something totally different. I try "listen" to my body and if I feel I need some extra vitamin C I take some but I do not take it on a regular basis.

Iron

Prolonged aspirin use can lead to iron deficiency and anaemia.[44] It is unlikely that the salicylate in food leads to the same symptoms.

Potassium

Potassium, along with other electrolytes, are involved in the maintenance of normal pH balance, and work in conjunction with calcium and magnesium in the maintenance of normal muscle contraction and relaxation, and nerve transmission

Symptoms of potassium deficiency include fatigue, muscle pain and weakness (particularly of the lower limbs), loss of appetite, nausea, drowsiness, feelings of apprehension, excessive thirst, irrational behaviour, irregular heartbeat. A diet low in fresh fruits and vegetables but high in sodium can lead to a potassium deficiency. The other main route is via the use of diuretics and other drugs such as salicylates.[45]

Zinc

A study by Ambanelli et al showed that aspirin appeared to increase loss of zinc in the urine. The effect was noted within three days of starting to take aspirin.[46]

Supplements more generally

Do not assume you have a deficiency and begin taking any of the above in isolation from a good multi vitamin/mineral supplement—you could do yourself more harm than good. Virtually all vitamins and minerals rely on others to work effectively and it is possible to take in toxic doses so check with your doctor first.

Be cautious of information online. Whilst some health care practitioners recommend very high doses (in comparison to the recommended daily allowance) of vitamins for optimum health, many do not. What works for one person could, literally, be fatal for another. Take the middle way and be cautious.

A low salicylate diet can still provide all the vitamins and minerals that you need. If you are really worried about this as a possible problem do discuss it with your doctor. I suspect if any supplementation is needed it will most likely be additional vitamin C and a multi-vitamin and mineral but we are all different.

After my first few months on a low salicylate diet I began supplementing in therapeutic doses (large amounts) and saw some major changes including the healing of scars that were years old. I now only take small "maintenance" doses when I feel the need. I think I benefited from the high doses because my body had been ill for so long.

The challenge for a salicylate sensitive is to find supplements that are salicylate and salicylate mimic free. Avoid any with added colours, flavourings, and preservatives. Check and double check and treat them all as suspect—by this I mean you should test them like you would a food. Start by taking one of your chosen supplements for a number of days and monitor your reactions. If you experience any adverse reactions then stop taking them. I have had reactions to all types of supplements with vitamin E and fish oils being the worst.

I have tried various brands and now only buy from either Solgar or BioCare but that may change in the future depending on how the companies manufacture their supplements. Unfortunately, ingredients used do change, sometimes with alarming regularity, so I am not going to recommend any particular supplement as I have no way of knowing which will be safe for salicylate sensitives when you read this book.

Do not assume that vitamin and mineral supplements are safe. Many are laden with salicylate so check all labels carefully and if in doubt contact the manufacturer for more information—be warned not all of them understand what salicylate is or all the different ways in which it may be present

Key things to check for and avoid are added preservatives, colours, binders and fillers, herbs and vegetable extracts.

The safest method of dealing with vitamins and supplements of any type is to treat them as suspect. Introduce one you think is safe and carefully monitor your health over at least two weeks—if your salicylate level seems to have risen or you get unwanted symptoms and you know your overall intake of salicylate has been low then you must view the supplement as suspect. Remove it from your diet and monitor yourself for an improvement. I know it's tedious but it is far safer and, in the long term, easier to do it this way.

Vitamin C often comes from a plant source such as rose hips and this type may cause problems. Some types of vitamin E are derived from plants and these also may cause a problem. I have reacted to vegetable oils that have used vitamin E as an antioxidant rather than BHA or BHT and can only assume that the source of the vitamin E was the problem. I also experienced problems with what appear to be salicylate free cereals. Most commercial brands of these cereals contain a range of added vitamins—no information is provided on the source of these or whether they may have been treated with antioxidants or preservatives.

References

[1] Allen DH, Van Nunen S, Loblay R, Clarke L, Swain A. Adverse reactions to foods. Med J Aust 1984;141(5 Suppl):S37-42.

[2] Patriarca G, Venuti A, Schiavino D, Fais G. Intolerance to aspirin: clinical and immunological studies. Z Immunitatsforsch Immunobiol 1976;151(4):295-304.

[3] Lessof MH. Food intolerance. Scand J Gastroenterol Suppl 1985;109:117-21.

[4] Sainte-Laudy J. Acetylsalicylic acid: hypersensitivity, intolerance, or allergy? Allerg Immunol (Paris) 2001;33(3):120-6.

[5] Speer F, Denison TR, Baptist JE.. Aspirin allergy. Ann Allergy 1981;46(3):123-6.

[6] Szczeklik A. Aspirin-induced asthma. In: Aspirin and Other Salicylates. Ed Vane JR, Botting RM. Chapman and Hall 1992, 548-575.

[7] Cotton EK, Fahlberg VI. Hypoglycaemia with salicylate poisoning. A report of two cases. Am J Dis Children, 1964;108:171-3.

[8] Drummond R Nadine Kadri N, St-Cyr J. Delayed salicylate toxicity following enteric-coated acetylsalicylic acid overdose: a case report and review of the literature. Can J Em Med 2001;3(1).

[9] van Heijst ANP, van Dijk A. Acetylsalicylic acid (PIM 006). http://www.inchem.org/documents/pims/pharm/aspirin.htm

[10] Hartwig-Otto H. Pharmacokinetic considerations of common analgesics and antipyretics. Am J Med 1983 75 (suppl):30-7.

[11] Proudfoot AT. Toxicity of salicylates. Am J Med 1983;14:99- 103.

[12] Breakey J, Hill M, Reilly C, Connell H. Report of a trial of the low additive, low salicylate diet in the treatment of behaviour and learning problems in children. Aust J Nutr Diet 1991;48:89-94.

[13] Feingold B, Feingold H. The Feingold Cookbook for Hyperactive Children and others with problems associated with food additives and salicylates. 1979 Random House.

[14] Hertz-Picciotto I. Effects of aspirin on female reproductive function and on in utero development. In: Feinman S (ed). Beneficial and Toxic Effects of Aspirin. CRC Press 1994, 73-88.

[15] Higgs GA, Salmon JA. Is aspirin a pro-drug for salicylate? In: Aspirin and Other Salicylates. Ed Vane JR, Botting RM. Chapman and Hall 1992, 63-73.

[16] Dahlen B, Boreus LO, Anderson P, Andersson R, Zetterstrom O. Plasma acetylsalicylic acid and salicylic acid levels during aspirin provocation in aspirin-sensitive subjects. Allergy 1994;49(1):43-9.

[17] Temple AR, George DJ, Done AK, Thompson JA. Salicylate poisoning complicated by fluid retention. Clin Toxicol 1976;9:61-8.

[18] Miller CS. Are we on the threshold of a new theory of disease? Toxicant-induced loss of tolerance and its relationship to addiction and abdiction. Toxicol Ind Health 1999;15(3-4):284-94.

[19] Alberti A, Pirrone P, Elia M, Waring RH, Romano C. Sulphation deficit in "low-functioning" autistic children: a pilot study. Biological Psychiatry 1999;46(3):420-4.

[20] Bamforth KJ, Jones AL, Roberts RC, Coughtrie MW. Common food additives are potent inhibitors of human liver 17 alpha-ethinyloestradiol and dopamine sulphotransferases. Biochem Pharmacol 1993;46(10):1713-20.

[21] Baranczyk-Kuzma A, Sawicki J. Biotransformation in monkey brain: coupling of sulfation to glutathione conjugation. Life Sci 1997;61(18):1829-41.

[22] Scadding GK et al. Poor sulphoxidation ability in patients with food sensitivity. British Medical Journal 1988;297(6641):105-7.

[23] Raithel M, Baenkler HW, Naegel A, Buchwald F, Schultis HW, Backhaus B, Kimpel S, Koch H, Mach K, Hahn EG, Konturek PC. Significance of salicylate intolerance in diseases of the lower gastrointestinal tract. J Physiol Pharmacol. 2005 Sep;56 Suppl 5:89-102.

[24] Manning ME, Stevenson DD. Aspirin sensitivity. A distressing reaction that is now often treatable. Postgrad Med 1991;90(5):227-33.

[25] MacPherson CR, et al. The excretion of salicylate. Br J Pharmacol 1955;10:484-489. Smith PK. Studies on the pharmacology of salicylate. J Pharmacol Exp Ther 1946;87:237-255.

[26] Smith PK. Studies on the pharmacology of salicylate. J Pharmacol Exp Ther 1946;87:237-255.

[27] Prescott LF, Balai-Mood M, Critchley JAJH, Johnstone AF, Proudfoot AT. Diuresis or urinary alkalinisation for salicylate poisoning. Br Med J, 1982;285:1383-6.

[28] Brenner BE, Simon RR. Management of salicylate intoxication. Drugs 1982;24(4):335-40.

[29] Stevenson DD, Arroyave CM, Bhat KN, Tan EM. Oral aspirin challenges in asthamatic patiens: a study of plasma histamine. Clin Allergy 1976;6(5):493-505.

[30] Meredith TJ, Vale JA. Salicylate poisoning. In: Vale and Meredith Eds. Poisoning Diagnosis and Treatment. Update Books 1981; 97-103.

[31] Temple AR, George DJ, Done AK, Thompson JA. Salicylate poisoning complicated by fluid retention. Clin Toxicol 1976;9:61-8.

[32] Duggin GG. Combination analgesic-induced kidney disease: the Australian experience. Am J Kidney Dis. 1996 Jul;28(1 Suppl 1):S39-47.

[33] Healy E, Newell L, Howarth P, Friedmann PS. Control of salicylate intolerance with fish oils. Br J Dermatol. 2008 Dec;159(6):1368-9.

[34] Montenero AS. Drugs producing vitamin deficiencies. Acta Vitaminol Enzymol 1980;2(1-2):27-45.

[35] Binkley NC, Krueger DC et al: Vitamin K supplementation reduces the serum concentrations of under-gamma-carboxylated osteocalcin in healthy young and elderly adults. Am J Clin Nutr 2000;72:1523-1528.

[36] Joss JD, LeBlond RF. Potentiation of warfarin anticoagulation associated with topical methyl salicylate. Ann Pharmacother 2000;34(6):729-33.

[37] Treib J, Blaes F, Haass A, Ohlmann D, Pindur G, Hamann GF. Cerebral infarct in chronic acetylsalicylic acid poisoning. Nervenarzt 1996;67(4):333-4.

[38] Alonso-Aperte E, Varela-Moreiras G. Facultad de CC. Drugs-nutrient interactions: a potential problem during adolescence. Eur J Clin Nutr 2000;54 Suppl 1:S69-74.

[39] Buist RA. Drug-nutrient interactions:an overview. Intl Clin Nutr Rev 1984;4(3):114.

[40] Lawrence, VA. et al. Aspirin and folate binding: in vivo and in vitro studies of serum binding and urinary excretion of endogenous folate. J Lab.Clin Med 103:944-948, 1984.

[41] Inoue F, Walsh RJ. Folate supplements and phenytoin-salicylate interaction. Neurology 1983;33(1):115-6.

[42] Loh HS, Watters K, Wilson CW. The effects of aspirin on the metabolic availability of ascorbic acid in human beings. J Clin Pharmacol. 1973 Nov-Dec;13(11):480-6.

[43] http://www.umm.edu/altmed/articles/vitamin-c-000339.htm

[44] Leonards JR, Levy G, Niemczura R. Gastrointestinal blood loss during prolonged aspirin administration. N Engl J Med 1973;289(19):1020-2.

[45] Smith, MJH. and Smith, PK. eds. The Salicylates: A Critical Bibliographic Review. New York, Interscience, 1966.

[46] Ambanelli U, Ferraccioli GF, Serventi G, Vaona GL. Changes in serum and urinary zinc induced by ASA and indomethacin. Scand J Rheumatol 1982;11:63–4.

5 Survival Strategies

Living with a salicylate sensitivity is not always easy but it is possible. How difficult it becomes will vary tremendously from individual to individual. If you only react to salicylate in foods and medicines then things will be easier than if you also have reactions to airborne salicylate.

When the going gets tough, as at some point it will, remember how much better you feel now than you did before. The changes in health, physical and mental, can be profound but as time moves on it is easy to forget just what a difference they have made. I know that I often used to start the day in tears because my joints hurt so badly I could hardly get myself to the bathroom, that sinusitis was a constant misery of pain and balance problems, that I had a constant ringing in my ears, that my clothes would fit one day and not the next, my skin would change from looking good to awful. Just keep reminding yourself and as time moves on the new lifestyle will become more familiar and easier.

Tips and tricks to help you develop strategies for dealing with various aspects of salicylate sensitivity are given below.

Food

01. Get organised and plan ahead so that you always have food available that you can eat.

02. Use your freezer—make up extra batches of meals for the days when you just can't be bothered to cook or don't have time.

03. Never trust food given to you by others unless you know for definite that they understand what a salicylate sensitivity is. Even then you would be safest to check by asking for a full list of the ingredients.

04. Prepare a list of foods that you can eat (rather than ones you can't) that you can give to others or to restaurants to help them in preparing a meal for you.

05. If you are invited out for a meal always offer to bring some of your own food. Don't worry about offending your host—your offer could be a big relief.

06. If you are making a long journey always take more food and drink with you than you think you will need—unexpected delays can turn into nightmares if you don't have food and drinks with you that are safe for you.

07. Take time out to invent or discover new recipes—this will help you stop getting bored with the food you can eat.

08. If you buy any processed food, always check the ingredients as these do change.

09. Eat as balanced and varied a diet as you can.

10. If you deviate from your diet, either by choice or by necessity, do not give yourself a hard time. Learn from the experience and move on.

Airborne Salicylate

01. Eliminate as many potential sources of salicylate from within your home as you can.

02. Discuss your sensitivity with your employer and, if need be, ask to be moved to a better ventilated area or, if it all possible, to one that will remain free from salicylate laden products.

03. Ask your company, school, office to look into the possibility of using fragrance free cleaning products and establishing a fragrance free policy.

04. Consider whether you need to use an air filter.

05. Invest in a face mask for use in highly scented places.

06. Use your mask whenever you need to. I have at times had to put mine on at a checkout because of the perfume an assistant was wearing or because the surface had just been sprayed with a scented cleaning agent.

07. You will get stared at if you use a mask. People do not know why you are wearing one and are simply curious. In situations, like checkouts in shops and in banks, I explain as I am finding my mask that I am about to place one over my face because I have a perfume allergy which usually elicits concern and/or sharing of similar experiences.

08. Always have a shower immediately when you return home from a shopping or social trip and wash or "contain" clothing that has become contaminated with fragrances.

09. Go shopping at the quietest times of the day.

10. Don't become a hermit. There are lots of activities that do not need you to be closeted in a highly perfumed atmosphere.

Dealing with Reactions

01. Always remember that salicylate builds up in your body so that when you are looking for the cause of a reaction you may need to think back over a number of days.

02. If you are having difficulty identifying the source of your problems, keep a food diary that also records details of where you went and what you did.

03. Take the neutralising action that works for you, whether that be alkalising salts, increasing the amount of water you drink, lime juice, homeopathy or extra vitamin C, as soon as you can.

04. There will be times when things go wrong. Eating out whether at other peoples houses or restaurants is fraught with problems and sooner or later you will experience an unpleasant reaction. Learn from it and move on. Harsh advice? I don't think so. It is too easy to get locked into negative feelings about how restricted your diet is and maybe some of your activities. Best to simply do the best you can and focus on the positive—at least you know what went wrong and next time you will be able to avoid it.

05. If necessity places you in a situation where you have no control over your diet for a length of time then your body will once again adapt to the high salicylate. You will experience

problems but you will be able to cope. I would advice that, as soon as you can, you return to a low salicylate diet.

06. I suspect that some people who tried a low salicylate diet for themselves or their children have run into this problem— an improvement followed later by seemingly salicylate unrelated problems. The symptoms are the same as before but you know the tolerance level has not been exceeded. If this happens check your environment at work, home, school, wherever you spend time. Recheck all the food you have eaten especially for hidden ingredients such as colours, flavours and antioxidants.

General

01. Never assume that the person you are speaking to understands what salicylates are or what a salicylate sensitivity entails. This applies to everyone including health care workers, food chefs, and manufacturers of supplements.

02. If you ask a company to provide you with more information on a product make sure you also ask about additives and ask specifically about "non active" ingredients.

03. Use the term "allergic" rather than "food intolerant" with people you don't know—allergy is more accepted and most people will understand that this means you have a problem that needs to be taken seriously.

04. Never forget that what works for you may not work for anyone else—avoid trying to convert others and evangelising about the joys of additive free/low salicylate living. By all means do share your experience and explain your sensitivity but do know when to stop.

05. Don't expect understanding and support. Again, this is harsh advice but for your sanity it is best followed. Some people are very understanding, others simply are not and with some people it will not make any difference how much you explain or argue.

06. If you have relatives or friends who refuse to accept your sensitivity you will have to take control of where and when you see them. If you have to visit their homes then take your own food with you and keep doing this until they get the message (sadly, some never will). Chose to be assertive about your needs rather than taking on the victim role.

07. Take advice but then check it out for yourself—nobody has all the answers. The best expert on you, and your children, is always going to be you.

08. If reactions affect your mind, prepare to deal with them. Have strategies in place for avoiding contact, explaining your behaviour, making yourself feel safe. You may also find it useful, when well, to write yourself a note which you can read when a reaction takes hold—it should explain what is happening and reassure you that it will pass. If you have someone who understands what is happening talk to them as sometimes this helps minimise the effects of the anxiety.

09. Accept that your condition, whether understood by others or not, is serious and always look after yourself as best as you can.

10. Be gentle with yourself.

Other Food Problems

If you find that after initial improvement you continue to have some problems and are as certain as you can be that these are not being caused by salicylates then you may need to investigate other food problems. In an earlier chapter, I mentioned the difficulties that many salicylate sensitives have with wheat and milk. The other problem area for many is with other food chemicals most notably Amines, Monosodium Glutamate (MSG), and Solanine.

Amines

Amines are naturally occurring chemicals in certain foods which, like salicylates, are cumulative in the body. Over a period of time these can build up in your system causing reactions that mimic allergies. Amines are produced in food as a result of protein breakdown and/or fermentation which means they are often highly concentrated in processed foods.

Naturally occurring amines are generally thought to act in the body as neurotransmitters and the term "biogenic" amines is now frequently applied to these. These biogenic amines include amongst their number—histamine, phenylethylamine, serotonin and tyramine. Some people, however, seem to have a more general sensitivity to amines. Diets low in food chemicals usually include amines in this more general way.

Cooking certain foods, in particular meats, at high temperatures produces a set of amines that were not present before. One group of these is heterocyclic amines (HCAs). More than 17 different types of HCAs have been found in meat cooked at high temperatures. Stewing, barbecuing and frying appear to produce the most HCAs. Gravies made from meat juices, therefore, also have a high amine content.

Apparently, cooking in a microwave does not produce HCAs to anywhere near the same extent.

The other form of amine produced by cooking is polycyclic aromatic hydrocarbons (PAH). These are formed by the browning of carbohydrate based foods such as bread and are found in foods such as smoked and grilled meats and coffee. A sensitivity to these amines can often be misinterpreted as an intolerance specific to one type of food. For example, if toast doesn't agree with you it is easy to think that wheat is the problem; if a grilled steak upsets you then you might think you have a problem with beef.

Do not overcook food and always eat your food as fresh as possible. Pickling, smoking and other forms of preserving all increase the number of amines.

There is no specific list of symptoms indicated for amines but migraines that don't respond to other treatments may be relieved by a diet low in amines. The key to testing for an amine intolerance is to reduce the amount of amines in your diet, and hence your body, over a period of two weeks. Eliminate all the high and very high amine foods. Read the food lists carefully—if you are a regularly consumer of the foods in the moderate list reduce these also.

A way of keeping track of the amount of amines you are eating is to allocate each portion the number 1 and add these up each day. If you then find you have some improvement but not a lot you could reduce the amount of amines more easily in this way.

Re-think your cooking style. Avoid over cooking anything and avoid meat cooked in sauces as these will most likely have a high amine content. Never eat anything that has been burnt and avoid toasted breakfast cereals. After two weeks, eat some of the high and very high foods (only those low in salicylate) and monitor your response. Remember that amines are cumulative in the body.

Some people may immediately get a reaction such as a headache and others will only get similar symptoms after their level has increased—this can take up two weeks. Keep your food diary up to date and continue with scoring the number of amine portions you have had in any one day.

At the end of the testing time, if you have felt no better at all then you are unlikely to have an amine problem. If there has been a little improvement you may want to consider reducing your level even further and seeing if that increases the improvement.

If you have had a substantial improvement then you are amine sensitive and need to now work on establishing the level of amines you can generally tolerate. At this stage you may find your tolerance is very low but that over time this may change.

If you find you have a problem with amines do try alternative cooking methods before restricting your diet even further—many people find that their problems are only related to the amines produced by cooking methods.

Testing for amine content in food has been slow in taking place. The lists that follow are based on the available research but must not seen as the end of the story. Amine content will vary within the same food type as it is greatly affected by the ageing and cooking process. You are welcome to try foods not on the lists but so as not to confuse the results it would be advisable to treat them as suspect and only introduce them at a later stage when you can clearly determine what is happening. The categories of food are very low, low, moderate, high and very high.

Amines in food: Very Low

Fruit: Apple, apricot, blueberry, gooseberry, lime, peach, pear, rhubarb, strawberry.

Vegetables and legumes: Asparagus, cabbage, carrot, celery, corn, courgette, cucumber, french beans, green pea, lettuce, lima beans, onion, peppers, potato, radish, soya bean, turnip.

Nuts and seeds: Chestnut, horse chestnut, sunflower, pine nut, pistachio.

Condiments: Herbs and spices.

Dairy: Butter, cottage cheese, milk, ricotta cheese, plain yoghurt but as fresh as possible.

Sweets and sweeteners: Carob, golden syrup, maple syrup, sugar.

Beverages: Cow and goat milk, lemonade, soya milk, decaffeinated coffee.

Amines in food: Low

Fruit: Black currant, cherry, grapefruit, honeydew melon, mandarin, red currant.

Nuts and seeds: Almond, cashew, coconut, macadamia.

Meat, fish, and poultry: Chicken eggs, beef, chicken (no skin), fish (white), lamb, rabbit, turkey (no skin), veal.

Misc: Plain corn chips, plain potato crisps, tacos.

Amines in food: Moderate

Fruit: Dates, kiwi fruit, orange, passion fruit, paw paw, tangerine.
Vegetables: Broccoli, cauliflower, olives.
Nuts and seeds: Brazil, hazelnut.
Meat, fish, and poultry: Any meat, fish and poultry older than two days. Any frozen meat. Chicken liver and skin, salmon (tinned), tuna (fresh).
Condiments: Malt vinegar.
Beverages: Coffee, coffee substitutes, tea, decaffeinated tea, most herbal teas.

Amines in food: High

Fruit: Avocado, banana, fig, grapes, lemon, pineapple, plum, raspberry.
Vegetables: Aubergine, gherkin, mushroom, tomato.
Nuts and seeds: Pecan, walnut.
Meat, fish, and poultry: Bacon, hot dogs, frozen fish, gravy, ham, mackerel (tinned), meat juices, meat loaf, offal, pork, sardines (tinned).
Dairy: Mild cheeses.
Condiments: Meat extracts, soy sauce, vinegar, Worcestershire sauce.
Sweets and sweeteners: Cocoa, milk chocolate, white chocolate.
Beverages: All fruit juices.

Amines in food: Very High

Vegetables: Butternut, sauuerkraut, spinach.

Meat and fish and poultry: Any form of dried, pickled, salted, or smoked fish and meat. Anchovies, beef liver, fish roe, pies and pasties, processed fish products (such as fish fingers, cakes, and pastes), salami, sausages, tuna (tinned).

Dairy: Virtually all cheeses including brie, camembert, cheddar, cheshire, Danish blue, edam, emmental, gloucester, gouda, gruyere, jarlsberg, leicester, mozarella, parmesan, processed cheese, provolone, roquefort, stilton, swiss, wensleydale.

Sweets and sweeteners: Dark chocolate.

Condiments: Hydrolysed protein, miso, tempeh, yeast extracts.

Beverages: Chocolate flavoured drinks, cocoa, cola type drinks, orange juice, tomato juice, vegetable juices.

Monosodium Glutamate (MSG)

MSG, monosodium glutamate, is the sodium salt of a naturally occurring amino acid—glutamic acid. Glutamate is essential to life and is found in cells throughout our body. It occurs in two forms, naturally in food and as an added flavour enhancer. Most of the glutamate our bodies receives is in a "bound" form and is gradually released as enzymes digest the protein food that it is part of. MSG, on the other hand, is a form of "free" glutamate that is instantly available to us and it is too much of this type that can lead to problems.

The degree of sensitivity experienced depends on the individual. Some people can tolerate vast amounts, others find themselves shaking and in an anxiety state after very little. The toxic reactions experienced by some people are generally because of an overload of MSG in its form as a flavour enhancer.

MSG intensifies some flavours and lessens others. It is an ideal additive for food manufacturers to "adjust" the taste of highly processed food and you can, without realising it, be ingesting quite large amounts of MSG. Generally made from the fermentation of corn, sugar beets, or sugar cane, MSG is a potential problem for anyone with an intolerance of these foods.

MSG has been linked with a number of conditions. It has been found to bring on asthma in some individuals, angioedema of the face, hands and feet, urticaria, fatigue, and behaviour problems. Reactions are often delayed by many hours.

MSG does seem to set of an addictive response and hence cause food cravings. One of the difficulties with diagnosing if you have an MSG sensitivity is that it is often an ingredient that is hidden. You will need to follow the avoidance process very carefully.

To test for MSG sensitivity avoid all foods containing MSG both naturally and as an added flavour enhancer for at least five days. Test in two stages. During the first stage, eat some of the foods in which MSG occurs naturally and monitor your response. If there is no adverse reaction then continue to the second stage of testing. If you do have a reaction then return to a no MSG diet for five days and then continue to the second stage. During the second stage, eat one of the foods you would have eaten before that contains added MSG.

Some people react immediately on eating any MSG whilst for others it is dose related—whereas one meal containing MSG may cause no problems, a second meal followed by a snack food with high levels can produce the symptoms. It is a cumulative process—you may be able to eat it once a week but not over a number of days in succession. If a large, for you, amount of MSG is ingested it is possible that the initial reaction will be severe but of short duration. You should not be fooled into thinking this is the only reaction you will get. Monitor yourself carefully over the next few days and notice any additional changes such as bloating, rashes, mental confusion, false energy and headaches.

Foods in which MSG naturally occurs:

Apricot, broccoli, grape, green pea, meat extracts, mushroom, plum, prune, raisin, sultana, soy sauce, spinach, sweet corn, tomato, yeast extracts.

Cheese (especially blue vein, brie, camembert, gouda, gruyere, parmesan, roquefort).

Drinks in which MSG occurs:

Brandy, liqueur, port, rum, sherry, tomato juice, vegetable juice, wine.

Processed Foods:

Avoid those containing any of the above foods or drinks. Also check all of the following:

Snack foods such as flavoured crisps, chips, and tacos.

Soya products such as soy sauce, miso, tamari, and tempeh.

Sauces, gravy mixes, and stock cubes. Meat and yeast extracts, pastes and pates made from fish and meat.

Watch out for the additive MSG; it can be listed as MSG, Monosodium Glutamate or Flavour Enhancer 621. Check labels very carefully—MSG now creeps into foods as diverse as crisps and soup.

Hidden MSG

It is possible that each of the following may contain MSG:

Ingredients: Autolyzed yeasts, bouillon, barley malt, broth, calcium caseinate, flavourings (including those listed as natural), HVP (hydrolysed vegetable protein), HPP (hydrolysed plant protein), kombu extract, malt extract, seasonings, sodium caseinate, textured protein.

Restaurants and take outs: Beware! Many restaurants and fast food outlets sprinkle MSG onto fresh foods such as fruit salads to prevent browning.

Chinese food often uses MSG as an ingredient.

MSG is also often one of the hidden or "secret" ingredients in fast food.

Solanine

Solanine is a toxic alkaloid found in certain vegetables most notably potatoes. It probably acts as a preservative in the plants that works by making itself poisonous to fungi and bacteria and so preserving the life of the plant. It has been implicated in serious cases of food poisoning and has even resulted in death. A toxic dose will usually result in severe digestive upset and, possibly, trembling, weakness, breathing difficulties and paralysis.

Vegetables containing solanine are all members of the deadly nightshade family. Everybody should know that eating potatoes that are green is dangerous and should be avoided. Always ensure that your potatoes are thoroughly peeled with all the sprouting parts removed and if the potato is green throw it away. Solanine is not destroyed by heating.

Aside from the rather serious toxic aspect of solanine there is a lesser problem of sensitivity that effects certain individuals. Ordinarily the liver will break down solanine and help us dispose of it but in some individuals this is not the case and an excess of solanine leads to inflammation.

If you have any condition involving painful joints you might like to try a solanine free diet for a while—improvements can be dramatic. Identified symptoms include arthritis, confusion, drowsiness, gastrointestinal problems, hallucinations, migraine, painful joints, trembling, and skin problems.

Testing for a solanine problem is relatively straightforward as so few foods are involved. Simply eliminate them all from your diet for two weeks. If there is an improvement you will then have to decide as to whether you wish to test solanine rich foods or not. If there has been no change then solanine is not a problem for you.

Be cautious if you are still eating any processed food as potato starch creeps into products as diverse as soup, cakes and ice cream. The foods which contain solanine are:

Aubergine
Cayenne
Chilli
Green and red peppers
Paprika
Potato
Tomato.

This is a relatively easy test for salicylate sensitives as the only food on the list you are likely to be eating is potato. Keep a careful note in your food diary of how you are doing. Do remember that solanine builds up in the system and that testing may show no reaction for some days.

Non Food Products

It is impossible for me to list products that are salicylate free. Not only do the ingredients vary from country to country but they are changed by manufactures on a regular basis. It is also the case that not everyone reacts to the salicylate mimics so you will have to experiment and find what works for you. The following tips may help.

01. Avoid products that are scented, high in herbs or salicylate chemicals.

02. Be cautious with hypoallergenic products as these are often high in salicylate.

03. Treat any new product as something that needs to be tested. For example, if you are trying a new shampoo don't use it for the first time just before an important engagement—a skin rash will do nothing for your self esteem and an inhaled reaction could lead to brain fogging and will definitely not help you.

04. When you find products that work for you then keep in a reasonable supply so that, should the manufacturer change the ingredients, you have a safe supply whilst you find an alternative product.

05. For cleaning cuts and sores, I have not found a safe antiseptic but instead use vodka.

06. Vodka is also excellent for dealing with sore throats but only gargle if you want to stay sober! Colloidal silver can also be of benefit but not everyone is convinced by it.

07. A perfectly adequate substitute for toothpaste is sodium bicarbonate—just dip a damp toothbrush into the powder. There are also now ionic toothbrushes that don't need toothpaste.

08. Remember that product labels do not always list inactive ingredients.

09. Microfiber cloths and water, or water and either sodium bicarbonate or vinegar work very well as cleaning agents around the home.

10. Certain types of man made fibres can cause some people problems— try wearing only cotton.

11. New clothing has often been treated with chemicals— wash it before wearing.

The Future

It is quite possible that, in the future, you will be able to tolerate higher levels of salicylate ingested from food. To test whether your tolerance has improved increase the amount of salicylate in your diet gradually and keep a food diary (use the scoring guide in the earlier section to help you) so that you can monitor your progress.

A study by Paul et al found that food reactions in some individuals only took place when they had been using some form of aspirin.[1] If you have a history of taking these type of drugs, you may find that your tolerance of salicylate in food will improve over time.

Gibson and Clancy assessed the role played by dietary chemicals in chronic idiopathic urticaria by challenge testing after an exclusion diet. Re-testing individuals after a year indicated that most of those who tested positive to salicylate or benzoate retained their sensitivity.[2]

Some studies mention attempts to desensitise people, mainly aspirin sensitive asthmatics, to aspirin. I am uncertain as to how successful these attempts have been, especially in the long term, and given that there are always alternative drug treatments I believe it is safest to always avoid these drugs. Whether your sensitivity will decrease over time will depend on many factors such as the original cause (which we currently know little about), your age (some children seem to outgrow the condition), your general state of health, the type of medication you have taken in the past and are prescribed in the future, and so on.

Despite the difficulties of living with a salicylate sensitivity, I am seriously grateful that I now have an explanation for my problems. Do I find it frustrating? Yes. Limiting? Yes. Annoying? Yes. But life is so much easier knowing what the problem is because I can do something about it. By keeping my diet low in salicylate and avoiding as much other contact with salicylate as possible, I have a quality of life I could only watch others experience before. I hope your sensitivity will reduce over time but don't despair if it doesn't—enjoy the better health you have and spare a thought for the countless numbers of individuals who are still struggling and don't know why.

Low Salicylate Meals

A low salicylate diet can be daunting at first so I have included, in this section, some outlines of meals to help you get started. The real trick to low salicylate cooking is simplicity—keep meals plain and you won't go far wrong. If you want to be more creative, take recipes you like and eliminate the high salicylate ingredients, substituting low salicylate ingredients where possible.

Breakfast

Peeled pear, banana, and rice puffs (there are brands on the market that are just rice).

Banana and oat cakes (home made).

Porridge made with cashew nut milk or water or any milk you find safe.

Muesli: You need to mix your own. Buy grains in the form of flakes that you are okay with such as oats, rice, millet, buckwheat, barley. Combine them together. Add a few cashew nuts broken up and a chopped, peeled, pear.

Boiled, poached or scrambled eggs and whatever type of bread you can eat.

Fried breakfasts can consist of meat, eggs, and bread. The lack of tomatoes is a problem here but you can make your own variation of baked beans by cooking them in advance with celery and swede to make a sauce of sorts.

Pancakes or waffles with maple syrup.

Toast and any spread you can tolerate.

Lunch

Soups made with some variation of lentils, beans, potatoes, cabbage, leeks, celery, shallots, grains or rice noodles. For example: Leek and butter bean soup.

Sandwich pastes/dips made from beans such as chick peas.

Sandwiches using bread you can tolerate with any meat or bean spread. Add in lettuce or have a side salad of celery, cabbage and bean sprouts.

Omelettes or eggs in some other form.

Burgers and salad.

Baked potatoes with any safe filling (don't eat the skin on the potatoes).

Main Meals

Chicken, turkey, beef, pork, fish etc... with potatoes, pasta or rice, and vegetables that are tolerated.

Stir fried meals using meat, bamboo shoots, shallots, leeks, bean sprouts, cabbage. Served with rice or pasta or rice noodles.

Quiches made with eggs, milk (any), leeks and cheese (if okay).

Pasta and cheese.

Burgers either made from meat or beans/lentils.

Homemade fish cakes.

Fried eggs and homemade chips. If you can only use a cold pressed oil you will not be able to deep fat fry. Potatoes cut into small pieces, tossed in oil and roasted in the oven make a reasonable chip substitute.

Fried rice with pulses or meat and safe vegetables.

Vegetables:

Stir fried bamboo shoots, bean sprouts and the tiniest amounts of broccoli or carrot.

Cabbage, a few Brussels sprouts, peas, celery, green beans, leeks, swede, mung bean sprouts.

Side salads can be made from combinations of lettuce, beans, celery, cabbage, bean sprouts, cashew nuts, apple.

Desserts

Fruit salad—pears, banana, honeydew melon, golden delicious apple. Add tiny amounts of other fruit for variety.

Baked pears, pear (and apple) crumble, home made biscuits or cakes, yoghurt, if tolerated, chocolate, pancakes.

Snacks

Oatcakes (home made), home made biscuits, cashew nuts, safe fruits, chocolate, cheese if tolerated, plain yoghurt, rice cakes.

References

[1] Paul E, Gall HM, Muller I, Moller R. Dramatic augmentation of a food allergy by acetylsalicylic acid. J Allergy Clin Immunol 2000;105(4):844.

[2] Gibson A, Clancy R. Management of chronic idiopathic urticaria by the identification and exclusion of dietary factors. Clin Allergy 1980;10(6):699-704.

6 Evidence

The studies mentioned below, and at other points in this book, all deal with instances where salicylate, in some form, has been found to cause particular symptoms and/or conditions in certain individuals. For the sake of simplicity, and brevity, I have generally omitted studies that deny or refute such connections.

Angioedema

Urticaria and angioedema have been frequently linked with an aspirin intolerance (details of some of the studies can be found in the section on urticaria below).

Other forms of angioedema have also been noticed. Ghislain and Ghislain reported on a case of angioedema limited only to the nape of the neck.[1] The symptoms occurred every morning for fifteen days, two or three hours after taking aspirin. Interestingly enough the individual concerned had been taking the 100mg of salicylic acid per day for the previous two years. The symptoms abated when aspirin was stopped and re-emerged when napoxen was taken (cross reactivity between aspirin and NSAIDs is common).

Asthma

Aspirin induced asthma is a recognised condition and sufferers often have additional symptoms such as chronic sinusitis and nasal polyposis. It is also the case that some individuals with aspirin induced asthma also react to other substances such as tartrazine, sodium benzoate and parabens.[2,3] In one study it was found to be the second most common reaction after urticaria/angioedema.[4]

In 1991, Maning and Stevenson wrote that aspirin-induced hypersensitivity affects a substantial number of people, including 20% or more of asthmatic patients.[5] Symptoms are dramatically triggered after ingestion of aspirin or a nonsteroidal anti-inflammatory drug, and can persist even after the drug is discontinued.[6]

McDonald et al found that for 8 out of 42 patients with asthma but no history of sensitivity to aspirin had their asthma exacerbated when challenge tested with 640mg of aspirin.[7]

Park et al found that sodium salicylate can cause breathing problems for individuals sensitive to aspirin and tartrazine.[8]

Chudwin et al report on the case of a woman whose asthma was exacerbated after taking aspirin for Rheumatoid Arthritis. On challenge testing it was discovered that she developed urticaria as a reaction to tartrazine; and urticaria and respiratory problems when tested with salicylic acid and also choline magnesium trisalicylate.[9]

Menthol turned out to be the cause of a 40-year-old woman's asthma. The menthol causing the problems was present in toothpaste and sweets.[10]

Behaviour

In the 1970s, Dr Feingold linked hyperactivity and other behavioural problems with additives (especially colours and antioxidants) and some salicylate foods. His work formed the foundation for many future studies most of which seemed to be have been designed with the intention of disproving his work. The focus of many of theses studies was on a limited number of additives and rarely looked at the role of salicylates.

A 1999 review by Jacobson and Schardt of two dozen scientific studies found that food dyes and certain foods can adversely affect children's behaviour. "Denying that food ingredients can exacerbate ADHD or other behavioural effects reflects ignorance of the scientific research, and ignoring that research jeopardises children's well-being".[11] Many of the studies reviewed dealt more with additives than with salicylates so I am not going to go into detail here. If you are interested do visit the CSPI web site[12] from which you can access the report.

Salzman reports on a study in which 31 children with behavioural problems and learning difficulties were tested for sensitivity to salicylates, artificial colours and flavours. Eighteen had a positive response, and 15 of these were given the Australian Version of the Feingold KP diet. Of these fifteen, 93% improved in the areas of overactivity, distractability, impulsiveness and excitability. Other problems such as sleeping problems and bed wetting were also partially or completely resolved. Salzman concluded that the additive and salicylate elimination diet significantly affects behaviour.[13]

Swain et al found that 81 out of a group of 140 children with behavioural disorders experienced significant improvement following the elimination of certain foods and food additives.[14] Novembre et al reported on cases in which reactions to the food additives tartrazine and benzoate group led to a range of symptoms affecting the central nervous system including headaches, concentration and learning problems, depression and over activity.[15]

Cook and Woodhill developed a diet following Feingold's advice and used it with 15 hyperkinetic children.[16] The findings were that parents of 10 children were "quite certain" and those of three others "fairly certain" that their children's behaviour improved substantially with the diet and relapsed when the diet was not followed. Other studies have noted an improvement in children's behaviour, cognitive capacity, physical co-ordination and sleep,[17] and in hyperkinetic behaviour.[18]

Breakey presents details of a study using an Australian version of the Feingold diet (low additive/low salicylate) with 71 families.[19] Sixty two of these families experienced sufficient beneficial changes to want to continue with the diet. Thirty-five felt the changes were dramatic with improvements in behaviour, learning difficulties, sleep patterns and/or bedwetting.

Breakey et al found that 79.5% of 516 children with behavioural and learning problems when placed on a low additive/low salicylate diet showed some improvement. They concluded that additives and salicylates were not the cause of the behaviour problems rather that they aggravated the "underlying predisposition in susceptible children".[20] I can find no evidence to substantiate such a conclusion. In fact countless parents can attest to the fact that when their previously poorly behaved children are placed on a low salicylate and additive free diet, the behaviour problems simply disappear and only emerge if there is a deviation in the diet. These children have no inherent predisposition to behaviour problems except in the sense that their systems cannot tolerate certain chemicals which when ingested leads to poisoning and hence unwanted symptoms. It is not a psychological or emotional problem but a biochemical one.

Sadly, no studies that I am aware of have explored the role of salicylates and salicylate mimics on adult behaviour. We have to make the assumption that if they affect children in this way that they will also affect adults. However, anecdotal evidence (usually personal testimonies) indicate that adults of varying ages, after following a low salicylate diet, do experience improvement (often total) in the following symptoms:

Agoraphobia, anxiety, claustrophobia, concentration, confusion, co-ordination, delusions, depression, distorted vision and hearing, hyperactivity, irritability, mental exhaustion, memory problems, mood swings, needing to be alone, and over sensitivity to noise, smell, light and touch.

Autism Spectrum Disorder

Hyperactivity is often a condiiton that occurs in children with autism spectrum disorder (ASD) which has led to some parents using variations of the Feingold diet. Srinivasan notes that "Salicylates are a subgroup of phenols, and some parents notice that patients with autism have occassional problems with breakdown of phenols".[21]

Blood Sugar Problems

Wunsch et al looked at the influence of sodium salicylate on insulin secretion and blood glucose behaviour in 6 metabolic healthy persons and 9 type II-diabetics.[22] In both groups the sodium salicylate led to higher insulin levels. Seltzer noted that hypoglycaemia can be caused by salicylate.[23]

Raschke al describe a case of severe refractory (not readily yielding to treatment) hypoglycaemia which arose after using a topical salicylate to treat psoriasis. The man concerned was suffering from end-stage renal disease which will have undoubtedly affected the severity of his reaction but the authors note that, more generally, salicylate markedly impairs gluconeogenesis which is the synthesis of glucose from noncarbohydrate precursors such as amino acids—a process which takes place largely in the liver to maintain blood glucose levels.[24]

They also note that salicylate increases glucose utilisation which can result in hypoglycaemia. These blood sugar problems can lead to a range of symptoms including nausea, sweating, weakness, faintness, confusion, hallucinations, headache, cold sweats, hypothermia, irritability, bizarre behaviour and fainting.

Some salicylate sensitives may experience what is known as "reactive" hypoglycaemia which occurs after eating the food that has stimulated the pancreas to overproduce insulin. [I have also experienced this type of reaction to inhaled salicylates.]

Children and Salicylate

The ever increasing number of children being diagnosed as suffering from ADHD and other behavioural disorders is alarming. In the US[25]:

Approximately 9.5% or 5.4 million children, 4-17 years of age, were diagnosed with ADHD, as of 2007.

The percentage of children with a parent-reported ADHD diagnosis increased by 22% between 2003 and 2007.

Rates of ADHD diagnosis increased an average of 3% per year from 1997 to 2006 and an average of 5.5% per year from 2003 to 2007. [26]

Boys were more likely than girls to have been diagnosed with ADHD.

Rates of ADHD diagnosis increased at a greater rate among older teens as compared to younger children.

In 2003, 2.5 million children in the US took medications for ADHD.[27] As of 2007, 2.7 million young people between four and seventeen years of age (66.3% of those with a current diagnosis) were receiving medication treatment for the disorder.[28] Side effects can include loss of appetite, decreased growth, insomnia, and headaches.[29] A study in 2006 also highlighted concerns about the effects of medication on the heart.[30] As there is evidence that clearly links diet with these conditions in children, my personal view is that the first "treatment" to be explored should always be diet.

The diets that have met with the most success in treating ADHD are ones that are low in salicylate and low in additives or are additive free The one most widely known is the Feingold diet.

The details presented in this handbook are similar but not the same as the Feingold program. The Feingold diet eliminates virtually the same additives but only reduces salicylates in food to a limited extent. The list of foods that are classed as containing salicylate is extremely small and has never been extended to include more recent research. The diet, as it stands, has obviously been very successful for many children but for a child with salicylate sensitivity it may not go far enough.

The list of foods provided is very similar to one I first started with and I had some remarkable improvement but then went on to experience strange episodes and this sent me into a very confusing period of time. It began to seem as if I was reacting to a whole host of foods and my diet became extremely limited. It was only when I discovered the fuller list of salicylate containing foods and adjusted my diet accordingly that these problems went away. What seemed like extreme multiple food intolerance wasn't, I was simply experiencing problems from a build up of salicylate.

If you are a parent of a child with ADHD and follow the Feingold program with success and then find that your child begins to re-experience some problems, I suggest you follow the protocol as regards salicylate in food, outlined in this handbook, to see if a greater salicylate sensitivity is a problem. It is very much the case that salicylate tolerance varies from individual to individual and other salicylate foods may also need to be reduced in or eliminated from your child's diet.

Concern is expressed to me about the healthiness of a low salicylate diet for children. In all honesty it has to be one of the healthiest diets around—no junk food, no artificial colours or flavourings, home cooked meals... But what about the reduction in vegetables and fruit? Well before we get too carried away here firstly think about how many fruit and vegetables children on an "normal" diet eat. The answer, sadly, is very few. I would almost hazard to say that a child on a low salicylate diet will eat more fruit and vegetables—once they understand how much better they feel, children, including very young ones, will welcome foods that are safe for them.

Anyone concerned about adequate nutrition should see a dietician or nutritionist for advice—make sure you take a list of the foods your child can eat rather than those he or she must avoid.

The other concern is that children will be perceived as being different and feel set apart from others of their own age. The CSPI booklet *A Parent's Guide to Diet, ADHD, and Behavior* quotes an 11 year old as saying "I would rather be different because of what I eat than because of how I behave".[31] As an adult looking back I can echo those sentiments. I felt so excluded and confused as a child that being different solely because of what I ate would have been sheer bliss in comparison to the agonies I was daily enduring.

It is interesting that the medical establishment rather than being excited about Feingold's discovery that additives can affect behaviour and an exclusion diet can bring great health benefits set out to disprove his work. Most of the research that was carried out was in some way flawed but the damage was done and attention turned away from natural cures to drug treatment.

Rimland's overview of these studies found them to be seriously lacking. His observations on the flaws in many of these studies include the criticism that arbitrary negative conclusions were drawn as, in many of the studies, some children were found to react to additives.[32] The reality is that no studies have replicated Feingold's work—most focused on a few selected additives and rarely did they take into consideration the time factor involved in changes appearing or appreciate the cumulative effect of these substances. As a researcher, I have been shocked at the poor quality, reasoning and abuse of data that has taken place.

The suffering caused to children whose lives could be changed for the better by simple changes in their diet is not acceptable to me. Scientific research is needed and is essential but designing or bending research to fit a view is in my opinion morally criminal. My personal view is that any form of treatment that relies on changes in diet has to be safer than drug treatment and to ignore the potential benefits of dietary changes is totally unacceptable.

As a parent you may be met with disbelief not only from doctors and health care workers but also from family and friends. Do not despair, find support from other parents who have made similar discoveries as you and persevere. If you are able to bring about improvements in your child's health and their behaviour without having to use drugs then what greater gift could you, other than life itself, give them? So many drugs have side effects that a safer alternative has to be more acceptable and what could be simpler or more natural than a change in diet.

Thankfully, since I first wrote this section there has been some recognition of the problems caused by some food additives.

Pelsser et al used a few foods diet with children diagnosed with ADHD. They were exploring whether a change in diet had an impact on physical and sleep complaints. They found that there was a significant improvement in a number of symptoms including headaches, abdominal pain, unusual thirst, unusual perspiration, tiredness, stomach problems and sleeping problems. The diet was very restricted so it was not possible for the researchers to identify which foods or food chemicals had been causing the problems. They concluded that a strictly supervised restricted elimination diet is a valuable instrument to assess whether ADHD is induced by food but that the prescription of diets on the basis of IgG blood tests should be discouraged.[33]

A review of thirty five years of research on the links between diet and ADHD by Stevens et al concluded that there is a subgroup of children with ADHD who improve if artificial food colours are removed from their diet. Some children also seem to be sensitive to common non salicylate foods such as milk, eggs, and wheat, as well as salicylate containing foods.[34]

In 2007, McCann et al published their findings on the links between food additives and hyperactive behaviour in children.[35] They had carried out a randomised double-blinded, placebo controlled trial to test whether the intake of artificial food colours and additives affected children's behaviour. The tests involved children in two age groups: three year olds, and eight to nine year olds.

They found that a mix of additives commonly found in children's food could exacerbate hyperactive behaviours such as inattention, impulsivity, and overactivity. Behavioural changes were noted in children who had been diagnosed with hyperactivity and also in children who had not. The additives used in this study were:

E102 Tartrazine
E104 Quinoline yellow
E110 Sunset yellow
E122 Carmoisine
E124 Ponceau 4R
E129 Allura Red
E211 Sodium Benzoate

At last there was a study that proved the link between behaviour and additives, and had been carried out in a way that was acceptable to the establishment. The editor of *American Academy of Pediatrics Grand Rounds* commented as follows: "The overall findings of the study are clear and require that even we skeptics who have long doubted parental claims of the effects of various foods on the behaviour of their children, admit we might have been wrong".[36]

It was quite strange watching official bodies and food manufacturers rushing to accommodate findings that literally weeks before they would have denied as being possible. In the UK food manufacturers began to make changes very quickly and the momentum increased so that from July 2010 a, European Union wide, warning has to be placed on any food or soft drink that contains any of the six colours—the label must carry the warning "may have adverse effects on activity and attention in children". Action in various other countries is also taking place to try implement similar measures.

Dementia/Delirium

A study of salicylate intoxication amongst the elderly suggested that salicylate intoxication should be considered in all elderly patients with dementia and/or delirium.[37]

Eye Problems

Nystagmus (involuntary movement of the eyes) was improved after a diet avoiding artificial food colours, the preservatives BHA and BHT and some salicylate containing foods.[38] The same study indicated a potential link with strabismus (squints). Inoue and Walsh also reported on a case of nystagmus after aspirin treatment.[39]

Few other studies have been carried out that have looked at eye problems related to salicylate. Anecdotal evidence suggests that along with eye muscle disorders, blurred and impaired vision is experienced by some salicylate sensitives. A study by Valeri et al, on rabbits not humans, indicated that salicylate can accumulate in the cornea, lens and retina when aspirin is administered repeatedly.[40] The implications of this type of build up have not been explored.

Transient myopia occurred in a patient following ingestion of 2.7g acetylsalicylic acid.[41] Lee noted a case of a pimple type rash on the eyes that was linked with aspirin intolerance.[42] Kalinke and Wuthrich reported on a case of progressive pigmented purpura which was triggered by tartrazine.[43] Oedema of the lower eyelids was noted by Hanzlik and Presko.[44]

Gastrointestinal Symptoms

A study by Faulkner-Hogg et al found that some individuals with coeliac disease who did not wholly improve on a gluten free diet were sensitive to salicylate.[45] On testing, salicylate was found to provoke diarrhoea, headache, nausea and flatulence.

In a review of studies that examined the role of adverse food reactions in irritable bowel syndrome, Niec et al noted that the most common trait in the identified problem foods was a high salicylate content.[46]

Pearson diagnosed a severe salicylate sensitivity for one Crohn's patient.[47] Dooley et al found that duodenogastric reflux is increased after the use of aspirin.[48]

Aspirin, and NSAIDs, have been frequently linked with gastrointestinal side-effects including complications such as bleeding and perforation.[49] What is not perhaps known so well is that dyspepsia (pain or discomfort centred in the upper part of the abdomen), often known as chronic indigestion, is a common side effect.[50] Salicylate in food can lead to similar symptoms for some individuals.

Prolonged use of salicylate led to 20% of the doctors participating in a British trial discontinuing use of aspirin because of dyspepsia and constipation.[51]

Whittle in his review of the unwanted effects of aspirin on the gastrointestinal tract concludes that evidence exists to "confirm that chronic use of aspirin and other non-steroid anti-inflammatory agents gives rise to serious toxic actions in the gastrointestinal tract including haemorrhage and ulcers in a large proportion of the patient population".[52] The potential benefits of using these drugs should be weighed against the potential side effects which could lead to additional treatment being necessary.

Hearing Difficulties

Salicylate is known to cause reversible hearing loss and tinnitus. It interferes with the outer hair cells which are believed to underlie normal hearing frequency, selectivity and sensitivity.[53]

Tinnitus is an accepted symptom of salicylate toxicity as has been frequently shown in various studies.[54] For example, Brien's review of toxicity associated with salicylates links tinnitus and hearing loss, usually reversible, with acute intoxication and long term administration of salicylates such as aspirin.[55]

And, Cazals notes that tinnitus may be the first subjectively recognised symptom of salicylate toxicity and presents evidence going back to 1877 which shows links between salicylates and tinnitus.[56] The dose of salicylate medications for the treatment of rheumatoid arthritis was often set below the point at which the individual started to experience tinnitus. Cazals found that salicylate could lead to tinnitus, sound distortion, deterioration of speech understanding and hypersensitivity to noise.

Although these studies have focused on manufactured forms of salicylate there is also evidence that dietary salicylate, in a sensitive individual, may also lead to tinnitus. In 1989 deBartolo reported that, over a twelve year period, they had identified individuals who are sensitive to salicylates and have improved or relieved their tinnitus with a salicylate free diet.[57] Shulman, in his book on the diagnosis and treatment of tinnitus, includes one of the potential triggers as being foods high in salicylate.[58]

Noise sensitivity as a reaction to salicylate intolerance has been noted.[59,60] Halla and Hardin found that tinnitus or subjective hearing loss or both were reported by 61 of 134 patients (45%) who were taking regular salicylates for rheumatoid arthritis. On measuring salicylate levels they were not able to identify a level at which these symptoms occur.[61] This does not surprise me as salicylate tolerance levels will vary greatly from individual to individual. It is also the case that the hearing problems are unlikely to have been constant in their severity—fluctuation in the severity of symptoms seems to correspond to fluctuating salicylate levels.

Joint Problems

One area of great improvement experienced by many individuals following a low salicylate diet is a reduction in joint and muscle pain.

It seems that salicylate-like drugs limit the formation of prostaglandins by interfering with cyclo-oxygenese activity. Vane and Botting's review of these effects left them with a question unanswered: is it beneficial to inhibit prostaglandin production in chronic inflammatory states? They note that one of the consequences could be the enhancement of cartilage breakdown.[62] If this does happen then one of the effects of too much salicylate will probably be joint pain and must raise questions about its use in the treatment of arthritis.

Kidney Problems

Acetylsalicylic acid has led to impaired kidney function, electrolyte imbalance, oedema, and nephrotoxicity in some individuals.[63]

Migraine

Migraine was found to be triggered by aspirin in aspirin sensitive asthmatics.[64]

Pancreatatitis

Cases in which 5-aminosalicylic acid has been used as part of drug treatment for conditions such as ulcerative colitis have led to the development of pancreatitis for some individuals.[65]

Rhinitis/Sinusitis/Polyps

Intolerance to aspirin has been found to trigger rhinitis, sinusitis, nasal polyposis and asthma.[66]

Aspirin sensitive rhino sinusitis occurs more commonly in adults than children. Further sensitivities are often developed to substances such as tartrazine and food additives.[67]

Gosepath et al identified aspirin intolerance in patients with chronic sinusitis as a cause of early recurrence of the symptoms (including nasal polyposis) after surgical treatment in some patients.[68] Richtsmeier noted that some cases of chronic sinusitis are associated with aspirin allergy.[69]

Skin Complaints

Ballmer-Weber reported on a case of a 55 year old who suffered from recurrent episodes of generalised pustulosis and high temperatures which doctors eventually (after 4 years) discovered was being caused by a reaction to acetylsalicylic acid (aspirin).[70]

Lee et al describe the case of a 21-year-old woman who had been taking several kinds of pain relief medication for menstruation pains and developed a burning sensation on unexposed areas of her upper chest and back where, eight months earlier, she had sustained severe sunburn. It was found that the use of Bufferin (the main ingredient of which is aspirin) was the cause of this reaction.[71]

Calnan describes six cases of contact dermatitis, which spread in a ring around the mouth, from a lip salve; five of the people were found to be allergic to phenyl salicylate.[72] Other instances of contact dermatitis caused by phenyl salicylate have also been reported.[73,74] Severe atopic dermatitis has also been noted.[75]

Sonnex and Rycroft report on three cases of allergic contact dermatitis behind the ears from wearing the same brand of industrial safety spectacles. In two of the cases the problem substance was phenyl salicylate.[76]

Holmes and Freeman present the case of a 26-year-old woman who had suffered with persistent dermatitis of the lips for over 12 months. Despite cosmetic avoidance and various treatments her condition persisted. It was not until she experienced an acute reaction at the dentists to a mint-flavoured tooth cleaning powder that the problem was identified as being caused by mint and mint flavourings. Once she stopped using a mint flavoured toothpaste the problem ceased.[77]

Shelley describes the case of a six-year-old boy with generalised pustular psoriasis (psoriasis characterised by pus-like blisters on the skin usually on the hands or feet) due to a sensitivity to salicylates found in trees, shrubs, and medicines. The attacks were triggered by the chewing of birch leaves and twigs, and teaberry leaves (all very high in natural salicylate).[78]

Urticaria

A study by Speer et al showed that the most common manifestation of adverse reactions to aspirin is urticarica/angioedema.[79] Diez found that symptoms of intolerance to aspirin included angioedema and urticaria as did Settipane[80] and Speer[81]. Ortolani et al found 21% of a patient group with chronic urticaria-angioedema were intolerant to benzoic acid. They also noted a high incidence of cross reactivity to aspirin.[82] Botey et al present evidence of six children with urticaria and/or angioedema related to acetylsalicylic acid.[83]

Doeglas found that some individuals with chronic urticaria were aspirin sensitive, challenge tests always brought about urticaria. For most of these individuals reactions also took place to one or more of the following: tartrazine, sodium benzoate, 4-hydroxybenzoic acid, sodium- and phenyl salicylate and the analgesics indomethacin, paracetamol and mefanamic acid.[84] Recurrent urticaria in both children and adults has been noted.[85] Swain et al found that 86 out of 140 children with recurrent urticaria improved significantly on a salicylate free diet.[86]

Juhlin et al examined the sensitivity of aspirin-intolerant patients to p-hydroxybenzoate and sodium benzoate by oral provocation testing—urticaria was induced in 5 of 7 sufferers.[87]

Lindemayr and Schmidt found that urticaria, for some individuals, could be triggered by p-hydroxybenzoic acid propylester, benzoic acid, sodium benzoate, tartrazine, ponceau rouge and indigo carmine. Using a diet that avoided salicylates, benzoates and colours, 20% of those in the study recovered spontaneously and became symptom-free, a further 55% showed marked improvement.[88]

Wright and Minford described the case of a 23-month-old girl with chronic urticaria resistant to antihistamine therapy. Large quantities of a topical salicylate preparation were being regularly applied to her pacifier. Once this habit was stopped, her urticaria cleared and did not recur.[89]

Genton et al found that in some instances of urticaria the trigger was acetylsalicylic acid and/or tartrazine. Avoiding these for just 5 days usually resulted in marked improvement.[90]

Others

Loss of co-ordination and sleep disturbance.[91]

Exercise induced anaphylaxis: Dohi et al found that for some individuals aspirin exacerbated the risk of exercise induced anaphylaxis. They found that, of those studied, aspirin might be enhancing the release of histamine from mast cells whilst exercising.[92]

Mouth burns: Aspirin has been found to be the culprit for burns in the mouth of some individuals.[93,94]

Vomiting, lethargy and hyperpnea were caused in a 21 month old child after ingesting methyl salicylate (oil of wintergreen) in the form of candy flavouring.[95]

Prolonged use of salicylate containing tablets for headaches led a 60 year old woman being admitted to hospital in an abnormally drowsy state. Her symptoms leading up to this state included increasing weakness, tiredness, memory and speech disorders and tinnitus.[96]

Salicylate intoxication may occur through placental transfer[97] and breast milk[98].

References

[1] Ghislain PD, Ghislain E.Aspirin-induced angioedema of the nape of the neck with naproxen cross-reaction: a case report. Ann Med Interne (Paris) 2000;151(3):227-9.

[2] Sakakibara H, Suetsugu S. Aspirin-induced asthma as an important type of bronchial asthma. Nihon Kyobu Shikkan Gakkai Zasshi 1995;33 Suppl:106-15.

[3] Speer F. Aspirin allergy: a clinical study. South Med J 1975;68(3):314-8.

[4] Speer F, Denison TR, Baptist JE.. Aspirin allergy. Ann Allergy 1981;46(3):123-6.

[5] Manning ME, Stevenson DD. Pseudoallergic drug reactions: aspirin, nonsterodial anti-inflammatory drugs, dyes, additives and preservatives. Immunol. Alll Clin NA 1991:11:659.

[6] Manning ME, Stevenson DD. Aspirin sensitivity. A distressing reaction that is now often treatable. Postgrad Med 1991;90(5):227-33.

[7] McDonald JR, Mathieson CA, Stevenson DD. Aspirin intolerance in asthma: Detection by oral challenge. J Allergy 1972;50:198.

[8] Park HS et al. Sodium salicylate sensitivity in an asthmatic patient with aspirin sensitivity. J Korean Med Sci 1991;6(2):113-7.

[9] Chudwin DS, Strub M, Golden HE, Frey C, Richmond GW, Luskin AT. Sensitivity to non-acetylated salicylates in a patient with asthma, nasal polyps, and rheumatoid arthritis. Ann Allergy 1986;57(2):133-4.

[10] dos Santos MA, Santos Galvao CE, Morato Castro F. Menthol-induced asthma: a case report. J Investig Allergol Clin Immunol 2001;11(1):56-8.

[11] Jacobson MF, Schardt D. Diet, ADHD & Behavior: A Quater-Century Review. Center for Science in the Public Interest 1999.

[12] http://www.cspinet.org/

[13] Salzman LK. Allergy testing, psychological assessment and dietary treatment of the hyperactive child syndrome. Med J Aust 1976;2(7):248-51.

[14] Swain A, Soutter V, Loblay R, et al. Salicylates, oligoantigenic diets, and behaviour. Lancet 1985;2:41-42.

[15] Novembre E, Dini L, Bernardini R, Resti M, Vierucci A . Unusual reactions to food additives. Pediatr Med Chir 1992;14(1):39-42.

[16] Cook PS, Woodhill JM. The Feingold dietary treatment of the hyperkinetic syndrome. Med J Aust 1976;2(3):85-8, 90.

[17] Fitzsimon M, Holborow P, Berry P, Latham S. Salicylate sensitivity in children reported to respond to salicylate exclusion. Medical Journal of Australia 1978;2(12):570-2.

[18] Brenner A. A study of the efficacy of the Feingold diet on hyperkinetic children. Some favorable personal observations. Clin Pediatr (Phila) 1977;16:7:652-6.

[19] Breakey J. Dietray Management of Hyperkinesis and Behavioural Problems. Aus Fam Phy 1978;7:720-4.

[20] Breakey J, Hill M, Reilly C, Connell H. Report of a trial of the low additive, low salicylate diet in the treatment of behaviour and learning problems in children. Aust J Nutr Diet 1991;48:89-94.

[21] Srinivasan, P. A Review of dietary interventions in autism. Ann. Clin. Psych. 21:4, Nov. 2009, 237-247.

[22] Wunsch C, Lohmann D, Verlohren HJ. Effect of sodium salicylate on insulin secretion and blood glucose behavior in metabolically healthy and type II diabetic patients. Dtsch Z Verdau Stoffwechselkr 1985;45(6):317-24.

[23] Seltzer HS. Drug-induced hypoglycemia. A review of 1418 cases. Endocrinol Metab Clin North Am 1989;18:1:163-83.

[24] Raschke R, Arnold-Capell PA, Richeson R, Curry SC. Refractory hypoglycemia secondary to topical salicylate intoxication. Arch Intern Med 1991;151(3):591-3.

[25] http://www.cdc.gov/ncbddd/adhd/data.html

[26] Diagnosed Attention Deficit Hyperactivity Disorder and Learning Disability: United States, 2004–2006. CDC Vital and Health Statistics Series 10, No.237, July 2008.

[27] Stevens LJ, Kuczek T, Burgess JR, Hurt E, Arnold LE. Dietary sensitivities and ADHD symptoms: thirty-five years of research. Clin Pediatr (Phila). 2011 Apr;50(4):279-93.

[28] http://www.cdc.gov/ncbddd/adhd/data.html

[29] Stevens LJ, Kuczek T, Burgess JR, Hurt E, Arnold LE. Dietary sensitivities and ADHD symptoms: thirty-five years of research. Clin Pediatr (Phila). 2011 Apr;50(4):279-93.

[30] Nissen SE. ADHD drugs and cardiovascular risk. N Engl J Med. 2006;354:1445-1448.

[31] CSPI booklet 'A Parent's Guide to Diet, ADHD, and Behavior', 1991.

[32] Rimland B. The Feingold Diet: An Assessment of the Reviews by Mattes, by Kavale and Forness and others. J Learning Dis 1983;16(6):331-333.

[33] Pelsser LM, Frankena K, Toorman J, Savelkoul HF, Dubois AE, Pereira RR, Haagen TA, Rommelse NN, Buitelaar JK. Effects of a restricted

elimination diet on the behaviour of children with attention-deficit hyperactivity disorder (INCA study): a randomised controlled trial. Lancet. 2011 Feb 5;377(9764):494-503.

[34] Stevens LJ, Kuczek T, Burgess JR, Hurt E, Arnold LE. Dietary sensitivities and ADHD symptoms: thirty-five years of research. Clin Pediatr (Phila). 2011 Apr;50(4):279-93.

[35] McCann D, Barrett A, Cooper A, Crumpler D, Dalen L, Grimshaw K, Kitchin E, Lok K, Porteous L, Prince E, Sonuga-Barke E, Warner JO, Stevenson J. Food additives and hyperactive behaviour in 3-year-old and 8/9-year-old children in the community: a randomised, double-blinded, placebo-controlled trial. Lancet. 2007 Nov 3;370(9598):1560-7.

[36] Editor. ADHD and Food Additives revisited. AAP Grand Rounds. 2008; 19:17.

[37] Bailey RB, Jones SR Chronic salicylate intoxication. A common cause of morbidity in the elderly. J Am Geriatr Soc 1989;37(6):556-61.

[38] Feingold BF. Dietary management of nystagmus. J Neural Transm 1979;45:2:107-15.

[39] Inoue F, Walsh RJ. Folate supplements and phenytoin-salicylate interaction. Neurology 1983;33(1):115-6.

[40] Valeri P, Romanelli L, Martinelli B, Guglielmotti A, Catanese B. Time-course of aspirin and salicylate in ocular tissues of rabbits. Lens Eye Toxic Res 1989;6(3):465-75.

[41] Sandford-Smith JH.. Transient myopia occurred in a patient following the ingestion of 2.7g of aspirin. Br J Opthal,1974;58:698.

[42] Lee SG, Matsuyoshi N, Ohta K, Horiguchi Y, Imamura S. Drug eruption due to Bufferin showing erythema exsudativum multiforme with a photo-recall-like phenomenon. Eur J Dermatol 1998;8(4):280-2.

[43] Kalinke DU, Wuthrich B. Purpura pigmentosa progressiva in type III cryoglobulinemia and tartrazine intolerance. A follow-up over 20 years. Hautarzt 1999;50(1):47-51.

[44] Hanzlik PJ, Presko E. The salicylates. XIV. J Pharmacol 1923, 21: 247-61.

[45] Faulkner-Hogg KB, Selby WS, Loblay RH, Morrow AW. . Dietary analysis in symptomatic patients with coeliac disease on a gluten-free diet: the role of trace amounts of gluten and non-gluten food intolerances. Scand J Gastroenterol 1999;34(8):784-9.

[46] Niec AM, Frankum B, Talley NJ. Are adverse food reactions linked to irritable bowel syndrome? Am J Gastroenterol 1998;93(11):2184-90.

[47] Pearson M, Teahon K, Levi AJ, Bjarnason I. Food intolerance and Crohn's disease. Gut 1993;34(6):783-7.

[48] Dooley CP, Mello WD, Valenzuela JE. Effects of aspirin and prostaglandin E2 on interdigestive motility complex and duodenogastric reflux in man. Dig Dis Sci 1985;30(6):513-21.

[49] Lanas A. Cyclo-oxygenase-1/cyclo-oxygenase-2 non selective non-steroidal anti-inflammatory drugs: epidemiology of gastrointestinal events.Dig Liver Dis 2001;33 Suppl 2:S29-34.

[50] Nandurkar S, Talley NJ, Xia H, Mitchell H, Hazel S, Jones M. Dyspepsia in the community is linked to smoking and aspirin use but not to Helicobacter pylori infection. Arch Intern Med 1998;158(13):1427-33. Comment: ACP J Club. 1999;130(1):19.

[51] Peto R, Gray R, Collins R, et al. Randomised trial of prophylactic daily aspirin in British male doctors. Br Med J 1988; 296:313-6.

[52] Whittle BJR. Unwanted effects of aspirin and related agents on the gastrointestinal tract. In: Aspirin and Other Salicylates. Ed Vane JR, Botting RM. Chapman and Hall 1992, 465-509.

[53] Kakehata S, Santos-Sacchi J. Effects os Salicylate and Lanthanides on Outer Hair Cell Motility and Gating Charge. J Neurosc 1996;16(16):4881-89.

[54] Bauer CA, Brozoski TJ, Holder TM, Caspary DM. Effects of chronic salicylate on GABAergic activity in rat inferior colliculus. Hear Res 2000;147(1-2):175-182.

[55] Brien J A, Sigma. Ototoxicity associated with salicylates: A brief review. Drug Saf 1993;9(2):143-8.

[56] Cazals Y. Auditory sensori-neural alterations induced by salicylate. Prog Neurobiol 2000;62(6):583-631.

[57] DeBartolo H M Jr. Zinc and diet for tinnitus. Am Journal Otol 1989;10(3):256.

[58] Shulman, A. Tinnitus: Diagnosis/Treatment. Lea & Febiger, 1991.

[59] Chen CS, Aberdeen GC. Potentiation of acoustic-trauma-induced audiogenic seizure susceptibility by salicylates in mice. Experientia 1980;36(3):330-1.

[60] Chen CS, Aberdeen GC. Potentiation of noise-induced audiogenic seizure risk by salicylate in mice as a function of salicylate-noise exposure interval. Acta Otolaryngol 1980;90(1-2):61-5.

[61] Halla JT, Hardin JG. Salicylate ototoxicity in patients with rheumatoid arthritis: a controlled study. Ann Rheum Dis 1988;47(2):134-7.

[62] Vane JR, Botting RM. The Prostaglandins. In: Aspirin and Other Salicylates. Ed Vane JR, Botting RM. Chapman and Hall 1992, 17-34.

[63] Zambraski EJ, Dunn MJ. Renal effects of aspirin. In: Aspirin and Other Salicylates. Ed Vane JR, Botting RM. Chapman and Hall 1992, 510-530.

[64] Grzelewska-Rzymovska I, Bogucki A, Szmidt M. Migraine in aspiirin-sensitive asthmatics. Allergol Immunopathol 1985;13:13-16.

[65] Isaacs KL, Murphy D. Pancreatitis after rectal administration of 5-aminosalicylic acid. J Clin Gastroenterol 1990;12(2):198-9.

[66] Casterline CL. Intolerance to aspirin. Am Fam Physician 1975;12(5):119-22.

[67] Schapowal AG, Simon HU, Schmitz-Schumann M. Phenomenology, pathogenesis, diagnosis and treatment of aspirin-sensitive rhinosinusitis. Acta Otorhinolaryngol Belg 1995;49(3):235-50.

[68] Gosepath J, Hoffmann F, Schäfer D,. Amedee RG, Mann WJ. Aspirin Intolerance in Patients with Chronic Sinusitis. ORL 1999;61:3:146-150.

[69] Richtsmeier WJ. Medical and surgical management of sinusitis in adults. Ann Otol Rhinol Laryngol Suppl 1992;155:46-50.

[70] Ballmer-Weber BK, Widmer M, Burg G. Acetylsalicylic acid-induced generalized pustulosis. Schweiz Med Wochenschr 1993;123(12):542-6.

[71] Lee SG, Matsuyoshi N, Ohta K, Horiguchi Y, Imamura S. Drug eruption due to Bufferin showing erythema exsudativum multiforme with a photo-recall-like phenomenon. Eur J Dermatol 1998;8(4):280-2.

[72] Calnan CD. Cronin E. Rycroft RJ Allergy to phenyl salicylate. Contact Dermatitis. 1981;7(4):208-11.

[73] Fimiani M, Casini L, Bocci S. Contact dermatitis from phenyl salicylate in a galenic cream. Contact Dermatitis 1990;22(4):239.

[74] Sonnex TS, Rycroft RJ. Dermatitis from phenyl salicylate in safety spectacle frames. Contact Dermatitis 1986;14(5):268-70.

[75] Van Bever HP, Docx M, Stevens WJ. Food and food additives in severe atopic dermatitis. Allergy 1989;44(8):588-94.

[76] Sonnex TS, Rycroft RJ. Dermatitis from phenyl salicylate in safety spectacle frames. Contact Dermatitis 1986;14(5):268-70.

[77] Holmes G, Freeman S. Cheilitis caused by contact urticaria to mint flavoured toothpaste. Australas J Dermatol 2001;42(1):43-5.

[78] Shelley WB. Birch Pollen and Aspirin Psoriasis: A Study in Salicylate Hypersensitivity. JAMA 1964, 28;189:985-8.

[79] Speer F, Denison TR, Baptist JE.. Aspirin allergy. Ann Allergy 1981;46(3):123-6.

[80] Settipane GA. Aspirin and allergic diseases: a review. Am J Med 1983;74(6A):102-9.

[81] Speer F. Aspirin allergy: a clinical study. South Med J 1975;68(3):314-8.

[82] Ortoloni C, Pastorello E, Luraghi MT, Della Torre F, Bellani M, Zanussi C. Diagnosis of intolerance to food additives. Ann Allergy 1984;53:587-91.

[83] Botey J, Navarro C, Aulesa C, Marin A, Eseverri JL. Acetyl salicylic acid induced-urticaria and/or angioedema in atopic children. Allergol Immunopathol (Madr) 1988;16(1):43-7.

[84] Doeglas HM. Reactions to aspirin and food additives in patients with chronic urticaria, including the physical urticarias. Br J Dermatol 1975;93(2):135-44.

[85] Settipane RA, Constantine HP, Settipane GA. Aspirin intolerance and recurrent urticaria in normal adults and children. Epidemiology and review. Allergy 1980;35(2):149-54.

[86] Swain A , Dutten SP, Truswell AS. Salicylates in Food. J Am Dietetic Assoc 1985;85(8).

[87] Juhlin L, Michaelsson G, Zetterstrom O. Urticaria and asthma induced by food-and-drug additives in patients with aspirin hypersensitivity. J Allergy Clin Immunol 1972;50:92-98.

[88] Lindemayr H, Schmidt J.Intolerance to acetylsalicylacid and food additives in patients suffering from recurrent urticaria. Wien Klin Wochenschr 1979;91(24):817-22.

[89] Wright AL, Minford A. Urticaria and hidden salicylates. Pediatr Dermatol 1999;16(6):463-4.

[90] Genton C, Frei PC, Pecoud A. Value of oral provocation tests to aspirin and food additives in the routine investigation of asthma and chronic urticaria. J Allergy Clin Immunol ;76(1):40-5.

[91] Fitzsimon M, Holborow P, Berry P, Latham S. Salicylate sensitivity in children reported to respond to salicylate exclusion. Medical Journal of Australia 1978;2(12):570-2.

[92] Dohi M, Suko M, Sugiyama H, Yamashita N, Tadokoro K, Okudaira H, Ito K, Miyamoto T. 3 cases of food-dependent exercise-induced anaphylaxis in which aspirin intake exacerbated anaphylactic symptoms. Arerugi 1990;39(12):1598-604

[93] Dellinger TM, Livingston HM. Aspirin burn of the oral cavity. Ann Pharmacother 1998;32(10):1107.

[94] Kawashima Z, Flagg RH, Cox DE. Aspirin-induced oral lesion: report of case. J Am Dent Assoc 1975;91(1):130-1.

[95] Howrie DL, Moriarty R, Breit R Candy flavoring as a source of salicylate poisoning. Pediatrics 1985;75(5):869-71.

[96] Gogoll L, Bentsen P, Hochrein H. Cerebral complications in chronic acetylsalicylic acid poisoning. Dtsch Med Wochenschr 1989;114(5):177-80.

[97] Lynd PA, Andreasen AC, Wyatt RJ. Intrauterine salicylate intoxication in a newborn. Clin Pediatrics 1976 15:912-3.

[98] Clark JH, Wilson WG. A 16-day-old breast-fed infant with metabolic acidosis caused by salicylate. Clin Pediatr 1981;20:53-4.

Thank You

My thanks reach out to all the researchers, doctors, nurses, dieticians, and laboratory staff who have, over the years, carried out research into the effects of salicylates. Without their work many of us would be very ill and never know why. So, thank, thank you, thank you.

My gratitude also extends out to the countless individuals who have shared their stories over the years with me. You have helped me feel less alone and have made me feel proud to be part of a group of people who often strike me as being quite amazing. I have often been moved to tears by the struggles that individuals have gone through, have been amazed at the courage and strength shown when misdiagnosis has led to horrendous consequences, have been filled with admiration at your ability to keep on going, and have been honoured that so many of you have found comfort in my words. May health always, always be yours.

My thanks also extend to Alex, my husband, who knew me before I understood what salicylate sensitivity was. Thank you for always believing in me.

Appendix 1

Health Benefits of Aspirin

There rarely seems a month that passes without the benefits of aspirin as a preventative for some disease or the other making the news. Over the years, aspirin has been praised for its anti-inflammatory properties and been said to reduce the risks of developing heart disease and several types of cancer. Whilst it does appear to be the case that aspirin, for some individuals, is beneficial the news reports rarely mention the problems and potential side effects of regular long-term aspirin use.

As I was working on the new edition of this handbook, the press was full of articles on how regular aspirin dosage led to a reduced risk of colon cancer. The headlines would have had you convinced that aspirin worked to prevent cancer in everyone and that it was totally safe. The potential side effects and risks of taking the drug on a daily basis aside, what did the research actually find? For some individuals who were carriers of hereditary colorectal cancer (Lynch syndrome), a daily dose of 600 mg aspirin for a mean of 25 months substantially reduced cancer incidence after 55•7 months.[1] There is no way of knowing, from this one study, whether aspirin can prevent colon cancer more generally and it must never be forgotten that it is a drug and that it does, potentially, have serious side effects.

We keep hearing about these type of studies, so should we be worried that our salicylate levels are low and we could never take aspirin?

As the active chemical in aspirin is salicylic acid, some researchers have looked into whether naturally occurring salicylate in food can have the same effects within the body as taking larger doses in the form of aspirin. One of the problems that faces researchers is that we still have no single method of determining how much salicylate we generally take in from our food. The estimated daily intakes have ranged from 0.4 to 200mg/day.[2] The "benefits" attributed to aspirin have led to speculation on the role of salicylate in the diet and much discussion about salicylate deficiency. This concept of being deficient in salicylate is a relatively new one and arguments are put forward on two assumptions: firstly, that salicylate is essential for health and that it is obtained from the diet or from medication. Duthie and Wood point out that the identified protective effects of aspirin may have led to an over-emphasis on the importance of dietary salicylates with little regard to the other bioactive phenols that occur in plants rich in salicylate.[3]

We do not know if salicylic acid is essential for health. The idea that it is has arisen from the protective role assigned to aspirin in heart disease and prevention of certain cancers. The argument goes as follows:

- Aspirin is used extensively to reduce cardiovascular disease risk.
- There is some evidence that aspirin may reduce the risk of other chronic diseases such as certain forms of cancer.
- Salicylate is present naturally in fruits and vegetables and individuals with a low intake of these foods may be

"salicylate deficient". One solution would be to give people low doses of aspirin.[4]

Salicylic acid seems to capture some peoples imaginations as being a cure all and absolutely essential for health. There have even been calls to have salicylic acid classed as a vitamin with the name "Vitamin S".[5]

It has generally been thought that the salicylic acid that can be measured in humans is as a result of salicylate that has been ingested via food. Yet, it is possible that we produce salicylates or chemicals very similar to them. As Butriss explains, hydroxybenzoic acid derivatives, also known as phenolic acids, include benzoic acid and derivatives such as salicylic acid. Whilst benzoic acid can be obtained from the diet it can also be formed within the body from B-oxidation of 3-phenylpropionic acid which is a gut flora metabolite of tyrosine in humans.[6]

A 2008 study by Paterson et al found that salicylic acid was present in the body even if no dietary or medicine based salicylate had been ingested, This led them to speculate that salicylic acid was, at least partially, an endogenous compound: i.e. it was created within the body.[7]

A fascinating hypothesis but what concerns me about the study is that it did not take into account sources of salicylic acid that may have been inhaled or absorbed through the skin. However, if their findings prove to be correct then anyone with a salicylate sensitivity need never worry about lacking in the protective aspects of salicylic acid as the body will, regardless of your diet, produce some. Could it be possible that some of us produce too much? Without further research to confirm the hypothesis that we produce salicylic acid ourselves we have know way of knowing.

My personal view is that aspirin is too easily hailed as a cure or preventive agent and I suspect that this partially happens because the drug is readily available and cheap. I think because it can be bought over the counter in most shops we forget that it is a drug that can be harmful to some people and if taken in excess can kill. We also mustn't forget that there are side effects linked with aspirin use. A recent, 2011, study linked aspirin use with degenerative eye disease,[8] and the risks of gastrointestinal bleeding from even low dosage aspirin taken on regular basis are well known.[9,10,11] Duthie and Wood point out that with therapeutic doses of salicylic acid of 75mg a day there is "a peptic ulcer incidence of 5-10% over 3-6 months of usage, a bleeding complication rate of 0.5-2.0 per 100 patient years and a mortality rate of ulcer complications of about 5% of those who have been admitted to hospital due to ulcer bleeding".[12] They add that the risk of gastrointestinal toxicity from salicylate levels in food is probably low but do note that one study found aspirin intakes as low as 10mg a day causing gastric damage in humans.

So ignore the studies and headlines about how aspirin is essential for this condition or that disease. It is not going to do you any good reading them as you are not able to take aspirin. If you have specific concerns about heart disease or some hereditary condition then discuss the options that are open to you with a doctor—aspirin is rarely the only solution or option.

References

[1] http://www.thelancet.com/journals/lancet/article/PIIS0140-6736(11)61049-0/abstract

[2] Wood A, Baxter G, Thies F, Kyle J, Duthie G. A systematic review of salicylates in foods: estimated daily intake of a Scottish population. Mol Nutr Food Res. 2011 May;55 Suppl 1:S7-S14.

[3] Duthie GG, Wood AD. Natural salicylates: foods, functions and disease prevention. Food Funct. 2011 Sep 16;2(9):515-20.

[4] Morgan G. Should aspirin be used to counteract 'salicylate deficiency'? Pharmacol Toxicol. 2003 Oct;93(4):153-5.

[5] Morgan G. Could vitamin S (salicylate) protect against childhood cancer? Med Hypotheses. 2005;64(3):661.

[6] Buttriss J. Dietary Intake and Bioavailability of Plant Bioactive Compounds. In: Goldberg G (ed). Plants: Diet and Health (British Nutrition Foundation). Wiley-Blackwell, 2003.

[7] Paterson JR, Baxter G, Dreyer JS, Halket JM, Flynn R, Lawrence JR. Salicylic acid sans aspirin in animals and man: persistence in fasting and biosynthesis from benzoic acid. J. Agric Food Chem. 2008 Dec 24;56(24):11648-52.

[8] de Jong PT, Chakravarthy U, Rahu M, Seland J, Soubrane G, Topouzis F, Vingerling JR, Vioque J, Young I, Fletcher AE. Associations between Aspirin Use and Aging Macula Disorder The European Eye Study. Ophthalmology. 2011 Sep 13.

[9] Sostres C, Lanas A. Gastrointestinal effects of aspirin.Nat Rev Gastroenterol Hepatol. 2011 Jun 7;8(7):385-94.

[10] Sørensen HT, Mellemkjaer L, Blot WJ, Nielsen GL, Steffensen FH, McLaughlin JK, Olsen JH. Risk of upper gastrointestinal bleeding associated with use of low-dose aspirin. Am J Gastroenterol. 2000 Sep;95(9):2218-24.

[11] García Rodríguez LA, Lin KJ, Hernández-Díaz S, Johansson S.Risk of upper gastrointestinal bleeding with low-dose acetylsalicylic acid alone and in combination with clopidogrel and other medications. Circulation. 2011 Mar 15;123(10):1108-15.

[12] GG, Wood AD. Natural salicylates: foods, functions and disease prevention. Food Funct. 2011 Sep 16;2(9):515-20.

Appendix 2

Salicylate Chemicals

Some of the substances you need to watch out for are listed below. Please do be aware that this is not a comprehensive list of salicylate chemicals or salicylate mimics, it is rather a guide to show the types you need to be on the look out for and also to give you an idea of the vast range of such chemicals.

Some of the ones with the word salicylate or a derivative in their description:

5-aminosalicylic acid
5-Hydroxysalicylic acid
Acetylsalicylic acid
Acidium Salicylicum
Alkyl salicylate
Aluminium acetyl salicylate
Ammonium salicylate
Amyl salicylate
Antipyrin Salicylate
Benzyl salicylate
Bismuth subsalicylate
Buergeria salicifolia
Butyloctyl salicylate
Calcium salicylate

Menthyl salicylate
Methyl salicylate
Methylene disalicylic acid
Myristyl salicylate
Oxylsalicylate
Para-aminosalicylic acid
Pentyl salicylate
Phenyl salicylate
Phenethyl salicylate
Physostigmine salicylate
Potassium salicylate
Potassium amino salicylate
Procaine salicylate
Salactol

Calcium acetyl salicylate
Capryloyl salicylic acid
Chitosan salicylate
Choline salicylate
Cystamine bis-salicylamide
Dipropylene glycol salicylate
Eserine salicylate
Ethyl salicylate
Ethylhexyl salicylate
Glycol salicylate
Hexyldodecyl salicylate
Isoamyl salicylate
Isobutyl salicylate
Isocetyl salicylate
Isodecyl salicylate
Isopropyl salicylate
Lithium salicylate
Lythrum salicaria extract
Magnesium salicylate
Magsalyl
Mea-salicylate
Medocyoline sulfosalicylate

Sal ethyl carbonate
Salicare
Salicylaldehyde
Salicylamide
Salicylanilide
Salicylic acid
Salicylic alcohol
Saligen
Salipyrin
Salix alba bark extract
Salizylsaure
Salol
Salphenyl
Santyl (Santalyl salicylate)
Silanediol salicylate
Sodium salicylate
Stroncylate
Strontium salicylate
Sulfosalicylic acid
Thiosalicylic acid
Tridecyl salicylate
Trolamine salicylate

Other ingredients/products to be avoided without "salicylate" in their description:

2-hydroxybenzoic acid
2-hydroxybenzoic acid phenyl ester
2-hydroxybenzoic acid methyl ester
2-(methoxycarbonyl) phenol
2-Phenoxycarbonylphenol
Acido Orthoxibenzoico

Almond oil
Arthropan
Aspirin
Balsam of Peru
Balm Of Gilead
Benzaldehyde
Benzoate —any form
Benzoic acid
Beta Hydroxy Acid (BHA)
Beta hydroxy
Betula Oil
Birch
Bisabolol
Camphor
Carbolic acid
Castor oil
Cuplex
Direct Black 51
Duofilm
Ethoxybenzamide
Eugenol
Gentisic
Homosalate
Hydroxybenzoate
Hydroxybenzoic
Keralyt
Menthol
Mentholatum
Mesalamine Camphor
Mint
Monophytol
Musol
Myristyl

Oil of Gaultheria
Oil of wintergreen
Ortho-hydroxybenzoic acid
Peppermint oil
Phenazone
Phenic Acid
Phenol
Phenyl Alcohol
Populus nigra extract
Populus tremuloides extract
Pyralvex
Sodium 2-hydroxybenzoate acid
Stroncylate
Verrugon
Willow

Also ensure you avoid unsafe food additives and all herbs and spices—in cosmetics and toiletries these are often given their Latin name rather than their more common one so beware.

Index